# RYPINS' INTENSIVE REVIEWS

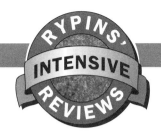

Series Editor

# Edward D. Frohlich, MD

Alton Ochsner Distinguished Scientist
Vice President for Academic Affairs
Alton Ochsner Medical Foundation
Staff Member, Ochsner Clinic
Professor of Medicine and of Physiology
Louisiana State University of Medicine
Adjunct Professor of Pharmacology and
Clinical Professor of Medicine
Tulane University School of Medicine
New Orleans, Louisiana

# RYPINS' INTENSIVE REVIEWS

# Psychiatry and Behavioral Medicine

## Gordon H. Deckert, MD, FACP

David Ross Boyd Professor
Department of Psychiatry and Behavioral Science
University of Oklahoma Health Sciences Center
Oklahoma City, Oklahoma

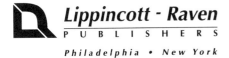

**Lippincott - Raven**
PUBLISHERS
*Philadelphia • New York*

Acquisitions Editor: Richard Winters
Sponsoring Editor: MaryBeth Murphy
Production Editor: Molly E. Dickmeyer
Design Coordinator: Melissa Olson
Managing Editor: Susan E. Kelly
Interior Designer: Susan Blaker
Cover Designer: William T. Donnelly
Production Service: P. M. Gordon Associates
Printer: Courier/Kendallville
Cover Printer: Lehigh Press

**Library of Congress Cataloging-in-Publication Data**

Deckert, Gordon H., 1930–
    Psychiatry and behavioral medicine / Gordon H. Deckert.
      p.  cm. — (Rypins' intensive reviews)
    Includes index.
    ISBN 0-397-51554-5
    1. Psychiatry — Outlines, syllabi, etc. 2. Psychiatry —
Examinations, questions, etc. I. Title. II. Series.
    [DNLM: 1. Mental Disorders — examination questions. 2. Behavioral
Medicine — examination questions.  WM 18.2 D295p 1997]
    RC457.2.D43  1997
    616.89' 0776 — dc20
    DNLM/DLC
    for Library of Congress          96-22473
                               CIP

9  8  7  6  5  4  3  2  1

Dedicated with gratitude
to mentors and colleagues too numerous to mention by name,
to thousands of students and residents now practicing medicine
    in every specialty,
to all those health professionals who attended workshops and
    presentations in and from every state in the Union,
to patients and to patients and to patients,
to fellow working members and staff of
    the National Board of Medical Examiners and
    the Federation of State Medical Examiners, and
    the Oklahoma Department of Health and its Board, and
    the University of Oklahoma,
but especially to three who have worked with me and beside me
    year after year after year—
    Jan Brewton, Departmental Secretary, now deceased,
    Beverly McKinney, Executive Secretary,
    Jane Chew Deckert, M.S., patient simulator extraordinary and
    partner forever.

## Who Was "Rypins"?

Dr. Harold Rypins (1892–1939) was the founding editor of what is now known as the RYPINS' series of review books. Originally published under the title *Medical State Board Examinations,* the first edition was published by J. B. Lippincott Company in 1933. Dr. Rypins edited subsequent editions of the book in 1935, 1937, and 1939 before his death that year. The series that he began has since become the longest-running and most successful publication of its kind, having served as an invaluable tool in the training of generations of medical students. Dr. Rypins was a member of the faculty of Albany Medical College in Albany, New York, and also served as Secretary of the New York State Board of Medical Examiners. His legacy to medical education flourishes today in the highly successful *Rypins' Basic Sciences Review* and *Rypins' Clinical Sciences Review,* now in their 16th editions, and in the *Rypins' Intensive Reviews* series of subject review volumes. We at Lippincott–Raven Publishers take pride in this continuing success.

—*The Publisher*

# ▼ Series Preface

These are indeed very exciting times in medicine. Having made this statement, one's thoughts immediately reflect about the major changes that are occurring in our overall healthcare delivery system, utilization-review and shortened hospitalizations, issues concerning quality assurance, ambulatory surgical procedures and medical clearances, and the impact of managed care on the practice of internal medicine and primary care. Each of these issues has had a considerable impact on the approach to the patient and on the practice of medicine.

But even more mind-boggling than the foregoing changes are the dramatic changes imposed on the practice of medicine by fundamental conceptual scientific innovations engendered by advances in basic science that no doubt will affect medical practice of the immediate future. Indeed, much of what we thought of as having a potential impact on the practice of medicine of the future has already been perceived. One need only take a cursory look at our weekly medical journals to realize that we are practicing "tomorrow's medicine today." And consider that the goal a few years ago of actually describing the human genome is now near reality.

Reflect, then, for a moment on our current thinking about genetics, molecular biology, cellular immunology, and other areas that have impacted upon our current understanding of the underlying mechanisms of the pathophysiological concepts of disease. Moreover, paralleling these innovations have been remarkable advances in the so-called "high tech" and "gee-whiz" aspects of how we diagnose disease and treat patients. We can now think with much greater perspective about the dimensions of more specific biologic diagnoses concerned with molecular perturbations; gene therapy not only affecting genetic but oncological diseases; more specific pharmacotherapy involving highly specific receptor inhibition, alterations of intracellular signal transduction, manipulations of cellular protein synthesis; immunosuppresive therapy not only with respect to organ transplantations but also of autoimmune and other immune-related diseases; and therapeutic means for manipulating organ remodeling or the intravascular placement of stents. Each of these concepts has become inculcated into our everyday medical practice within the past decade. The reason why these changes have so rapidly promoted an upheaval in medical practice is continuing medical education, a constant awareness of the current medical literature, and a thirst for new knowledge.

To assist the student and practitioner in the review process, the publisher and I have initiated a new approach in the publication of *Rypins' Basic Sciences Review* and *Rypins' Clinical Sciences Review*. Thus, when I assumed responsibility to edit this long-standing board review series with the 13th edition of the textbook (first published in 1931), it was with a feeling of great excitement. I perceived that great changes would be coming to medicine, and I believed that this would be one ideal means of not only facing these changes head on but also for me personally to cope and keep up with these changes. Over the subsequent editions, this confidence was reassured and rewarded. The presentation for the updating of medical information was tremendously enhanced by the substitution of new authors, as the former authority "standbys" stepped down or retired from our faculty. Each of the authors who continue to be selected for maintaining the character of our textbook is an authority in his or her respective area and has had considerable pedagogic and formal examination experience. One dramatic recent example of the changes in author replacement just came about with our forthcoming 17th edition. When I invited Dr. Peter Goldblatt to participate in the authorship of the pathology chapter of the textbook, his answer was "what goes around, comes around." You see, Dr. Goldblatt's father, Dr. Harry Goldblatt, a major contributor to the history of hypertensive disease, was the first author of the pathology chapter in 1931. What a satisfying experience for me personally. Other less human changes in our format came with the establishment of two soft cover volumes, the current basic and clinical sciences review volumes, replacing the single volume text of earlier years. Soon, a third supplementary volume concerned with questions and answers for the basic science volume appeared. Accompanying these more obvious changes was the constant updating of the knowledge base of each of the chapters, and this continues on into the present 17th edition.

And now we have introduced another major innovation in our presentation of the basic and clinical sciences reviews. This change is evidenced by the concurrent introduction of four volumes during this year representing four important chapters presented in the parent textbook: behavioral sciences, internal medicine, surgery, and psychiatry and behavioral medicine. Additional volumes, concerned with each of the other chapters of the parent textbook, will be published in subsequent years along with the 17th edition of *Rypins' Basic Sciences Review, Rypins' Clinical Sciences Review,* and the *Questions and Answers* third volume. These volumes are written to be used separately from the parent textbook. Each not only will contain the material published in their respective chapters of the textbook, but will be considerably "fleshed out" in the discussions, tables, figures, and questions and answers. Thus, we hope that the *Rypins' Intensive Reviews* series will serve as an important supplement to the overall review process and that it will also provide a study guide of those already in practice in preparing for specific specialty board certification and recertification examinations.

Therefore, with continued confidence and excitement, I am pleased to present these innovations in review experience for your consideration. As in the past, I look forward to learning of your comments and suggestions. In doing so, we continue to look forward to our continued growth and acceptance of the *Rypins'* review experience.

Edward D. Frohlich, MD, MACP, FACC

# ▼ Preface

Medical students enter medical school with at least 90% of their educational experience organized around what has been termed the **disciplinary assumption**. Here, the material is organized around a given body of knowledge that has its own internal set of logic. A good example is a textbook of biochemistry or a typical college course in economics or literature or zoology. This disciplinary organizing assumption continues and dominates the basic science years of medical school. Later, however, physicians discover that they simply cannot practice medicine within that organizational framework. Not that biochemistry or economics or psychology are not important. They are. But the disciplinary organizing assumption is simply not effective, and for several reasons.

Usually, the volume of material is overwhelming. So the brain "chunks" it. On average, short-term memory is capable of keeping five or six bits of information in mind at one time. It patterns it, and it looks for that pattern again and again when appropriately cued. When a given chunk does not fit a given perceptual or procedural reality at all, the information in the chunk is simply not used. Or, if there is a partial fit, information not there is inserted or assumed. The problem is that the organization of the material as presented is not in the format used by physicians of quality. By "physicians of quality" I mean those physicians operationally defined as more effective than their colleagues by outcome measures. Fortunately, many students "rechunk," usually during residency. But to the observation of attendings, pertinent information so often seems unavailable that some conclude clinicians should do all the basic science teaching. The counter from this discounted group is to discount: "Well, if you simply want this to be a trade school, go ahead." Both groups, in my opinion, are off the mark. On the other hand, clinicians often decide that somehow the students either were not taught or did not learn. "Where were you during your first two years of medical school?" or something like that is heard by almost every clerk sometime during his or her clinical years.

The second organizing assumption has been called the **subject assumption**. Here the material, the information, is organized around sets of subjects (patients, if you will) on whom this body of knowledge is to be visited. The standard design is around the theme of organ system nosology. Textbooks of internal medicine, psychiatry, orthopedics, pediatrics, and so on are almost exclusively organized in this fashion; all one need do is open their tables of contents and look. A similar design dominates the clinical years of medical school. Many physicians, some would say especially those in academic medical centers, never quite discover that it really is not possible to practice high-quality medicine exclusively or even primarily within this framework either!

There are understandable reasons for this. Patients do not come to a physician during a first illness encounter with the label "diabetes" stapled to their forehead. Usually, they do not even come suggesting that their physician turn to page 527, under Cardiovascular System Disease, to find a diagnostic explanation for their symptoms. Furthermore, most of those entities we call "diseases" are not limited to a single organ system. Also, particularly in the aging population, complaints, problems, and disabilities are usually the product of multiple diseases within and across interacting systems.

While I was flying to the West Coast to give a presentation, the gentleman sitting next to me said, "I'm guessing you are a professional." I acknowledged that was the case without specifying the profession, and asked him, "What is your field?" His reply was, "I'm a retinologist!" For a moment, I did not believe what I thought I heard. He did not say he was a physician specializing in ophthalmology, nor, for that matter, did he respond by saying he was an ophthalmologist specializing in the retina. He had taken a relatively small portion of the review of systems, a small chunk if you will, and made that his clinical identification. In my fantasy, I heard and saw him with a patient I called Mrs. Babcock. "Good morning, Mrs. Babcock." (Smiling) "It is good to meet you. Now shut up and let me look at your retina." I acknowledge this was my fantasy and may not be true of him at all. Yet, he does seem to say that he is an expert with retinas, and not an expert with people who have retinal disease.

There is a third organizational assumption, the **task assumption**. Here, the material, the experience, is not organized around a given disciplinary body of knowledge with its own internal set of logic, nor is it organized around the nosologic subject assumption. It is organized around the sequence of tasks that the practicing physician must use to have a therapeutic outcome with a specific patient. Not that nosology is insignificant to the practice of medicine. It is significant; in fact, it is critical. Paradoxically, it is so critical that it is important *not* to organize the learning experience predominantly within that frame. A major task for the reformation of medical education is understanding this concept and supporting it with an appropriate governance and an appropriate teaching and examining methodology.

The overall organizational assumption for this review is the task assumption. The review is organized around the sequence of tasks that the effective physician must perform to have a favorable outcome. Therefore, for the most part it does not read like a textbook. (Certain sections may—for example, the nosology section.) The goal for practicing physicians is to integrate a disease-oriented clinical practice with a patient-centered clinical practice with a population-based clinical practice. A summary of physician tasks is warranted by way of orientation to this review.

**Conceptual task.** Certain concepts that the physician brings to the patient encounter are critical to outcome. The biopsychosocial concept of dis-ease is one. This review goes beyond the concept to a biopsychosocial **model**—a way of thinking. It allows one to think simultaneously about biogenesis, psychogenesis, and sociogenesis. In the center stands the brain as a transducer. In the center stands the patient who is dis-eased, and in the center stands the disease. The model encourages diagnosis of the disease and diagnosis of the patient who is dis-eased.

**Attitudinal task.** This refers to how well the physician knows himself or herself. What are my psychological needs? How will they influence my practice of medicine, the way I deal with patients? Is this consistent with the professional role? Who am I today? How do I see my state of health? How am I feeling? How do I see my relationships with my significant others? What are my task pressures on this day? Knowing my psychological need profile and being familiar with today's psychological inventory prepares me, so to speak, for going to work. This task is not emphasized in this review. The reason is simple. You, the reader, are your own book; the answers to these questions must come from you.

**Perceptual task.** Perceptual skill is required for an effective patient-centered clinical practice. Considerable emphasis is given to nonverbal as well as verbal data. Because perception is a construction, it is important over time to know what I tend not to see and then learn to see it, what I tend not to hear and then learn to hear it. This requires a particular training, often self-imposed, because it is frequently missing in the formal training of medical school and residency. It is perfectly possible for a physician to practice for a lifetime and never discover the data he or she does not see or hear.

**Interpersonal task.** Accurate perception shapes the interactional task. The manner in which one proceeds with one patient is not the same as with another, even when the two share an identical, traditional, medical diagnosis. Physicians, as a group, have relatively mediocre communication skills. However, effective physicians possess and use specific and identifiable kinds of communication.

**Nosologic task.** The physician searches for an illness script, finds a relatively good match, and makes a diagnosis. Current *Diagnostic and Statistic Manual of Mental Disorders (DSM-IV)* nosology is outlined here with the nonpsychiatrist in mind. However, a traditional diagnosis is not enough. Emphasis is placed on diagnosing the patient in addition to the disease. Effective and experienced physicians place more reliance on instance scripts than on illness scripts. An instance script typically involves episodic memory more than semantic memory.

**Dynamic task.** Diagnosing the disease, although necessary, is not sufficient. Diagnosing the dis-ease, although required, is still not enough. Understanding the disease and the dis-ease in a specific patient requires modes of understanding. This review assumes some basic understanding of neuroanatomy, neurophysiology, neuropharmacology, the behavioral sciences, and one or more theories of psychodynamics.

**Therapeutic task.** The therapeutic sequence is emphasized. Therapy, for good or for ill, inevitably accompanies the evaluation process. It proceeds side by side with the physical examination, the writing of prescriptions, and the performance of procedures and treatment interventions.

Throughout this review, again and again, we will turn to what we know about the characteristics of effective physicians.

# ▼ Series Acknowledgments

In no other writing experience is one more dependent on others than in a textbook, especially a textbook that provides a broad review for the student and fellow practitioner. In this spirit, I am truly indebted to all who have contributed to our past and current understanding of the fundamental and clinical aspects related to the practice of medicine. No one individual ever provides the singular "breakthrough" so frequently attributed as such by the news media. Knowledge develops and grows as a result of continuing and exciting contributions of research from all disciplines, academic institutions, and nations. Clearly, outstanding investigators have been credited for major contributions, but those with true and understanding humility are quick to attribute the preceding input of knowledge by others to the growing body of knowledge. In this spirit, we acknowledge the long list of contributors to medicine over the generations. We also acknowledge that in no century has man so exceeded the sheer volume of these advances than in the twentieth century. Indeed, it has been said by many that the sum of new knowledge over the past 50 years has most likely exceeded all that had been contributed in the prior years.

With this spirit of more universal acknowledgment, I wish to recognize personally the interest, support, and suggestions made by my colleagues in my institution and elsewhere. I specifically refer to those people from my institution who were of particular help and are listed at the outset of the internal medicine volume. But, in addition to these colleagues, I want to express my deep appreciation to my institution and clinic for providing the opportunity and ambience to maintain and continue these academic pursuits. As I have often said, the primary mission of a school of medicine is that of education and research; the care of patients, a long secondary mission to ensure the conduct of the primary goal, has now also become a primary commitment in these more pragmatic times. In contrast, the primary mission of the major multispecialty clinics has been the care of patients, with education and research assuming secondary roles as these commitments become affordable. It is this distinction that sets the multispecialty clinic apart from other modes of medical practice.

Over and above a personal commitment and drive to assure publication of a textbook such as this is the tremendous support and loyalty of a hard-working and dedicated office staff. To this end, I am tremendously grateful and indebted to Mrs. Lillian Buffa and Mrs. Caramia Fairchild. Their long hours of unselfish work on my behalf and to satisfy their own interest in participating in this major educational effort is appreciated no end. I am personally deeply honored and thankful for their important roles in the publication of the Rypins' series.

Words of appreciation must be extended to the staff of the Lippincott–Raven Publishers. It is more than 25 years since I have become associated with this publishing house, one of the first to be established in our nation. Over these years, I have worked closely with Mr. Richard Winters, not only with the Rypins' editions but also with other textbooks. His has been a labor of commitment, interest, and full support—not only because of his responsibility to his institution, but also because of the excitement of publishing new knowledge. In recent years, we discussed at length the merits of adding the intensive review supplements to the parent textbook and together we worked out the details that have become the substance of our present "joint venture." Moreover, together we are willing to make the necessary changes to assure the intellectual success of this series. To this end, we are delighted to include a new member of our team effort, Ms. Susan Kelly. She joined our cause to ensure that the format of questions, the reference process of answers to those questions within the text itself, and the editorial process involved be natural and clear to our readers. I am grateful for each of these facets of the overall publication process.

Not the least is my everlasting love and appreciation to my family. I am particularly indebted to my parents who inculcated in me at a very early age the love of education, the respect for study and hard work, and the honor for those who share these values. In this regard, it would have been impossible for me to accomplish any of my academic pursuits without the love, inspiration, and continued support of my wife, Sherry. Not only has she maintained the personal encouragement to initiate and continue with these labors of love, but she has sustained and supported our family and home life so that these activities could be encouraged. Hopefully, these pursuits have not detracted from the development and love of our children, Margie, Bruce, and Lara. I assume that this has not occurred; we are so very proud that each is personally committed to education and research. How satisfying it is to realize that these ideals remain a familial characteristic.

Edward D. Frohlich, MD, MACP, FACC
New Orleans, Louisiana

# Introduction

# *Preparing for USMLE*

In August 1991 the Federation of State Medical Boards (FSMB) and the National Board of Medical Examiners (NBME) agreed to replace their respective examinations, the FLEX and NBME, with a new examination, the United States Medical Licensing Examination (USMLE). This examination will provide a common means for evaluating all applicants for medical licensure. It appears that this development in medical licensure will at last satisfy the needs for state medical boards licensure, the national medical board licensure, and licensure examinations for foreign medical graduates. This is because the 1991 agreement provides for a composite committee that equally represents both organizations (the FSMB and NBME) as well as a jointly appointed public member and a representative of the Educational Council for Foreign Medical Graduates (ECFMG).

As indicated in the USMLE announcement, "It is expected that students who enrolled in U.S. medical schools in the fall of 1990 or later and foreign medical graduates applying for ECFMG examinations beginning in 1993 will have access only to USMLE for purposes of licensure." The phaseout of the last regular examinations for licensure was completed in December 1994.

The new USMLE is administered in three steps. Step 1 focuses on fundamental basic biomedical science concepts, with particular emphasis on "principles and mechanisms underlying disease and modes of therapy." Step 2 is related to the clinical sciences, with examination on material necessary to practice medicine in a supervised setting. Step 3 is designed to focus on "aspects of biomedical and clinical science essential for the unsupervised practice of medicine."

Today Step 1 and Step 2 examinations are set up and scored as total comprehensive objective tests in the basic sciences and clinical sciences, respectively. The format of each part is no longer subject-oriented, that is, separated into sections specifically labeled Anatomy, Pathology, Medicine, Surgery, and so forth. Subject labels are therefore missing, and in each part questions from the different fields are intermixed or integrated so that the subject origin of any individual question is not immediately apparent, although it is known by the National Board office. Therefore, if necessary, individual subject grades can be extracted.

Step 1 is a two-day written test including questions in anatomy, biochemistry, microbiology, pathology, pharmacology, physiology, and the behavioral sciences. Each subject contributes to the examination a large number of questions designed to test not only knowledge of the subject itself but also "the subtler qualities of discrimination, judgment, and reasoning." Questions in such fields as molecular biology, cell biology, and genetics are included, as are questions to test the "candidate's recognition of the similarity or dissimilarity of diseases, drugs, and physiologic, behavioral, or pathologic processes." Problems are presented in narrative, tabular, or graphic form, followed by questions designed to assess the candidate's knowledge and comprehension of the situation described.

Step 2 is also a two-day written test that includes questions in internal medicine, obstetrics and gynecology, pediatrics, preventive medicine and public health, psychiatry, and surgery. The questions, like those in Step 1, cover a broad spectrum of knowledge in each of the clinical fields. In addition to individual questions, clinical problems are presented in the form of case histories, charts, roentgenograms, photographs of gross and microscopic pathologic specimens, laboratory data, and the like, and the candidate must answer questions concerning the interpretation of the data presented and their relation to the clinical problems. The questions are "designed to explore the extent of the candidate's knowledge of clinical situation, and to test his [or her] ability to bring information from many different clinical and basic science areas to bear upon these situations."

The examinations of both Step 1 and Step 2 are scored as a whole, certification being given on the basis of performance on the entire part, without reference to disciplinary breakdown. The grade for the examination is derived from the total number of questions answered correctly, rather than from an average of the grades in the component basic science or clinical science subjects. A candidate who fails will be required to repeat the entire examination. Nevertheless, as noted above, in spite of the interdisciplinary character of the examinations, all of the traditional disciplines are represented in the test, and separate grades for each subject can be extracted and reported separately to students, to state examining boards, or to those medical schools that request them for their own educational and academic purposes.

This type of interdisciplinary examination and the method of scoring the entire test as a unit have definite advantages, especially in view of the changing curricula in medical schools. The former type of rigid, almost standardized, curriculum, with its emphasis on specific subjects and a specified number of hours in each, has been replaced by a more liberal, open-ended curriculum, permitting emphasis in one or more fields and corresponding deemphasis in others. The result has been rather wide variations in the totality of education in different medical schools. Thus, the scoring of these tests as a whole permits accommodation to this variability in the curricula of different schools. Within the total score, weakness in one subject that has received relatively little emphasis in a given school may be balanced by strength in other subjects.

The rationale for this type of comprehensive examination as replacement for the traditional department-oriented examination in the basic sciences and the clinical sciences is given in the National Board Examiner:

The student, as he [or she] confronts these examinations, must abandon the idea of "thinking like a physiologist" in answering a question labeled "physiology" or "thinking like a surgeon" in answering a question labeled "surgery." The one question may have been written by a biochemist or a pharmacologist; the other question may have been written by an internist or a pediatrician. The pattern of these examinations will direct the student to thinking more broadly of the basic sciences in Step 1 and to thinking of patients and their problems in Step 2.

Until a few years ago, the Part I examination could not be taken until the work of the second year in medical school had been completed, and the Part II test was given only to students who had completed the major part of the fourth year. Now students, if they feel they are ready, may be admitted to any regularly scheduled Step 1 or Step 2 examination during any year of their medical course without prerequisite completion of specified courses or chronologic periods of study. Thus, emphasis is placed on the acquisition of knowledge and competence rather than the completion of predetermined periods.

Candidates are eligible for Step 3 after they have passed Steps 1 and 2, have received the M.D. degree from an approved medical school in the United States or Canada, and subsequent to the receipt of the M.D. degree, have served at least six months in an approved hospital internship or residency. Under certain circumstances, consideration may be given to other types of graduate training provided they meet with the approval of the National Board. After passing the Step 3 examination, candidates will receive their Diplomas as of the date of the satisfactory completion of an internship or residency program. If candidates have completed the approved hospital training prior to completion of Step 3, they will receive certification as of the date of the successful completion of Step 3.

The Step 3 examination, as noted above, is an objective test of general clinical competence. It occupies one full day and is divided into two sections, the first of which is a multiple-choice examination that relates to the interpretation of clinical data presented primarily in pictorial form, such as pictures of patients, gross and microscopic lesions, electrocardiograms, charts, and graphs. The second section, entitled Patient Management Problems, utilizes a programmed-testing technique designed to measure the candidate's clinical judgment in the management of patients. This technique simulates clinical situations in which the physician is faced with the problems of patient management presented in a sequential programmed pattern. A set of some four to six problems is related to each of a series of patients. In the scoring of this section, candidates are given credit for correct choices; they are penalized for errors of commission (selection of procedures that are unnecessary or are contraindicated) and for errors of omission (failure to select indicated procedures).

All parts of the National Board examinations are given in many centers, usually in medical schools, in nearly every large city in the United States as well as in a few cities in Canada, Puerto Rico, and the Canal Zone. In some cities, such as New York, Chicago, and Baltimore, the examination may be given in more than one center.

The examinations of the National Board have become recognized as the most comprehensive test of knowledge of the medical sciences and their clinical application produced in this country.

# THE NATIONAL BOARD OF MEDICAL EXAMINERS

For years the National Board examinations have served as an index of the medical education of the period and have strongly influenced higher educational standards in each of the medical sciences. The Diploma of the National Board is accepted by 47 state licensing authorities, the District of Columbia, and the Commonwealth of Puerto Rico in lieu of the examination usually required for licensure and is recognized in the American Medical Directory by the letters DNB following the name of the physician holding National Board certification.

The National Board of Medical Examiners has been a leader in developing new and more reliable techniques of testing, not only for knowledge in all medical fields but also for clinical competence and fitness to practice. In recent years, too, a number of medical schools, several specialty certifying boards, professional medical societies organized to encourage their members to keep abreast of progress in medicine, and other professional qualifying agencies have called upon the National Board's professional staff for advice or for the actual preparation of tests to be employed in evaluating medical knowledge, effectiveness of teaching, and professional competence in certain medical fields. In all cases, advantage has been taken of the validity and effectiveness of the objective, multiple-choice type of examination, a technique the National Board has played an important role in bringing to its present state of perfection and discriminatory effectiveness.

Objective examinations permit a large number of questions to be asked, and approximately 150 to 180 questions can be answered in a $2\frac{1}{2}$-hour period. Because the answer sheets are scored by machine, the grading can be accomplished rapidly, accurately, and impartially. It is completely unbiased and based on percentile ranking. Of long-range significance is the facility with which the total test and individual questions can be subjected to thorough and rapid statistical analyses, thus providing a sound basis for comparative studies of medical school teaching and for continuing improvement in the quality of the test itself.

# QUESTIONS

Over the years, many different forms of objective questions have been devised to test not only medical knowledge but also those subtler qualities of discrimination, judgment, and reasoning. Certain types of questions may test an individual's recognition of the similarity or dissimilarity of diseases, drugs, and physiologic or pathologic processes. Other questions test judgment as to cause and effect or the lack of causal relationships. Case histories or patient problems are used to simulate the experience of a physician confronted with a diagnostic problem; a series of questions then tests the individual's understanding of related aspects of the case, such as signs and symptoms, associated laboratory findings, treatment, complications, and prognosis. Case-history questions are set up purposely to place emphasis on correct diagnosis within a context comparable with the experience of actual practice.

It is apparent from recent certification and board examinations that the examiners are devoting more attention in their construction of questions to more practical means of testing basic and clinical knowledge. This greater realism in testing relates to an increasingly interdisciplinary approach toward fundamental material and to the direct relevance accorded practical clinical problems. These more recent approaches to questions have been incorporated into this review series.

Of course, the new approaches to testing add to the difficulty experienced by the student or physician preparing for board or certification examinations. With this in mind, the author of this review is acutely aware not only of the interrelationships of fundamental information within the basic science disciplines and their clinical implications but also of the necessity to present this material clearly and concisely despite its complexity. For this reason, the questions are devised to test knowledge of specific material within the text and identify areas for more intensive study, if necessary. Also, those preparing for examinations must be aware of the interdisciplinary nature of fundamental clinical material, the common multifactorial characteristics of disease mechanisms, and the necessity to shift back and forth from one discipline to another in order to appreciate the less than clear-cut nature separating the pedagogic disciplines.

The different types of questions that may be used on examinations include the completion-type question, where the individual must select one best answer among a number of possible choices, most often five, although there may be three or four; the completion-type question in the negative form, where all but one of the choices is correct and words such as *except* or *least* appear in the question; the true-false type of question, which tests an understanding of cause and effect in relationship to medicine; the multiple true-false type, in which the question may have one, several, or all correct choices; one matching-type question, which tests association and relatedness and uses four choices, two of which use the word, *both* or *neither;* another matching-type question that uses anywhere from three to twenty-six choices and may have more than one correct answer; and, as noted above, the patient-oriented question, which is written around a case and may have several questions included as a group or set.

Many of these question types may be used in course or practice exams; however, at this time the most commonly used types of questions on the USMLE exams are the completion-type question (one best answer), the completion-type negative form, and the multiple matching-type question, designating specifically how many choices are correct. Often included within the questions are graphic elements such as diagrams, charts, graphs, electrocardiograms, roentgenograms, or photomicrographs to elicit knowledge of structure, function, the course of a clinical situation, or a statistical tabulation. Questions then may be asked in relation to designated elements of the same. As noted above, case histories or patient-oriented questions are more frequently used on these examinations, requiring the individual to use more analytic abilities and less memorization-type data.

For further detailed information concerning developments in the evolution of the examination process for medical licensure (for graduates of both U.S. and foreign medical schools), those interested should contact the National Board of Medical Examiners at 3750 Market Street, Philadelphia, PA 19104, USA; telephone number 215–590–9500.

## FIVE POINTS TO REMEMBER

In order for the candidate to maximize chances for passing these examinations, a few common sense strategies or guidelines should be kept in mind.

First, it is imperative to prepare thoroughly for the examination. Know well the types of questions to be presented and the pedagogic areas of particular weakness, and devote more preparatory study time to these areas of weakness. Do not use too much time restudying areas in which there is a feeling of great confidence and do not leave unexplored those areas in which there is less confidence. Finally, be well rested before the test and, if possible, avoid traveling to the city of testing that morning or late the evening before.

Second, know well the format of the examination and the instructions before becoming immersed in the challenge at hand. This information can be obtained from many published texts and brochures or directly from the testing service (National Board of Medical Examiners, 3750 Market Street, Philadelphia, PA 19104; telephone 215–590–9500). In addition, many available texts and self-assessment types of examination are valuable for practice.

Third, know well the overall time allotted for the examination and its components and the scope of the test to be faced. These may be learned by a rapid review of the examination itself. Then, proceed with the test at a careful, deliberate, and steady pace without spending an inordinate amount of time on any single question. For example, certain questions such as the "one best answer" probably should be allotted 1 to $1\frac{1}{2}$ minutes each. The "matching" type of question should be allotted a similar amount of time.

Fourth, if a question is particularly disturbing, note appropriately the question (put a mark on the question sheet) and return to this point later. Don't compromise yourself by so concentrating on a likely "loser" that several "winners" are eliminated because of inadequate time. One way to save this time on a particular "stickler" is to play your initial choice; your chances of a correct answer are always best with your first impression. If there is no initial choice, reread the question.

Fifth, allow adequate time to review answers, to return to the questions that were unanswered and "flagged" for later attention, and check every $n$th (e.g., 20th) question to make certain that the answers are appropriate and that you did not inadvertently skip a question in the booklet or answer on the sheet (this can happen easily under these stressful circumstances).

There is nothing magical about these five points. They are simple and just make common sense. If you have prepared well, have gotten a good night's sleep, have eaten a good breakfast, and follow the preceding five points, the chances are that you will not have to return for a second go-around.

Edward D. Frohlich, MD, MACP, FACC

# Contents

# Chapter 1

# Biopsychosocial Concept of Disease

Medical students bring to medical school and physicians bring to their practice, whether they recognize it or not, a concept of what it is like to be a doctor, a concept of health and disease, a concept of what society expects the doctor to be and to do. These conceptual sets lead to certain consequences. What is it that is important for me to know? What should I learn? What skills should I develop? Can all activities of living organisms be explained in terms of their component molecular parts? Is the underlying principle of the practice of medicine physicochemical reductionism? Are all human health problems amenable to technological solutions? And later, what is it I first want to know when I see a patient? What are the characteristics of more effective physicians? How can I achieve a more favorable outcome?

## HISTORY

Humans are curious about themselves. They have always attempted to explain their behavior, including that behavior called mental illness. Humans have a tendency to ascribe the phenomena of mental illness to supernatural causes, especially to possession by some outside influence. Nonetheless, many early Greek physicians, including Hippocrates, taught that mental illness resulted from natural causes, and both Hippocrates and his near contemporary in India, Susruta, held a rather sophisticated view of psychosomatic processes. After the death of the Roman physician, Galen, in A.D. 200, a gradual return of primitive attitudes in the West culminated in demonology and the persecution and execution of so-called witches. This practice was much more pervasive in parts of Europe than is generally recognized. In the late 15th and early 16th centuries, conservative estimates put the figure of executions to approximately 100,000 in Germany and a similar number in France. *Malleus Maleficarum* (*The Witch's Hammer*), published by two Dominicans, Sprenger and Kramer, has had a profound influence on Western medicine. Western medicine's separation of mind from body during this time was perhaps inevitable given the theology of

*Rypins' Intensive Reviews: Psychiatry and Behavioral Medicine,* by Gordon H. Deckert. Lippincott–Raven Publishers, Philadelphia © 1997.

the day. Thomas Aquinas spoke for his culture and his age when he argued that the soul could not be sick. During this era, advances in medical psychology were found primarily in the Moslem world, especially among Arab physicians.

The first effective answer to demonology was *De Praestigüs Daemonum*, by Johann Weyer (1515–1588), often called "the father of psychiatry." Two centuries later in 1792, Philippe Pinel struck the chains from mental patients in the Bicetré in France. His contemporary, Benjamin Rush, a physician and a signer of the Declaration of Independence, was considered the father of American psychiatry because of his efforts on behalf of the mentally ill in Philadelphia.

During the 19th century, French and German psychiatrists, especially Emil Kraepelin (1855–1926), applied descriptive and statistical methods to clinical studies and elaborated a classification of personality disorders and mental illness. This classification still influences ours today. Later, Eugene Bleuler revisited the Kraepelinian concept of dementia praecox and introduced the term **schizophrenia**.

Paralleling the development of descriptive psychiatry was an increasing understanding of psychological mechanisms. Many scholars trace a sequence of ideas from Paracelsus (1493–1541) to Franz Anton Mesmer (1733–1815) to James Braid (1795–1860), who coined the term "hypnosis," to Jean Martin Charcot (1825–1893), among others, to the first giant in dynamic psychiatry, Sigmund Freud (1856–1939). His concepts of the unconscious; the ego, id, and superego; defense mechanisms; and neurotic conflict have become an integral part of psychiatric thought. Some of these terms are now used on an everyday basis by the public as well. His emphasis on early life experiences as a determinant of later behavior was one stimulus among many for the increasing interest in psychological growth and development, of which Jean Piaget's study of the development of the intellect is only one example. Modification of Freudian psychoanalytic theory to include broader sociologic and cultural influences is perhaps most prominently evident in the work of Erik Erikson.

More recently, a series of discoveries involving the brain and its neurophysiology and neurochemistry have reintegrated biology into modern psychiatry, along with descriptive (phenomenologic), psychological, sociologic, and cultural approaches. Today, when examining a given patient, the physician must be capable of thinking and working within these multiple frameworks of understanding human behavior, whether the behavior in question is molecular or molar. The term **biopsychosocial** is often used in this context.

# BEYOND THE BIOPSYCHOSOCIAL CONCEPT OF DISEASE

Scientists shape their models of explanation around the dominant metaphors of their time. In the 19th century, causes, processes, and effects were seen as linear. Electricity was compared to the flow of water. Infectious disease was simply caused by an organism invading an organism; psychopathology evolved when a trauma damaged a psyche—linear concepts of disease!

But in the 20th century and into the 21st, Einstein's relativistic field theory colors our metaphor. Today, we think in terms of systems, systems interacting with systems, multiple levels of organization within systems and between systems, and, more recently, with particular emphasis on the exchange of information across system boundaries. In 1977, Engel argued for a biopsychosocial approach to medical practice (Fig. 1-1).

The idea embodied in the neologism seemed to strike a resonant note within medicine: "My goodness, come to think of it, disease is not a thing after all. It is an event." Disease is a process, multiply determined interactively by biologic, psychological, and sociologic factors.

A biopsychosocial concept? Yes. But a model? A model implies a greater degree of operational specificity. Science uses the term "model" in at least three ways. First, a scientist may speak of a mathematical model. The second is exemplified in psychiatry by the lamentation that we do not possess a good animal model for schizophrenia. In the third sense, a model specifies a way of thinking—in our case, thinking about disease, diagnosing disease, dissecting its pathogenesis, and planning and implementing interventions.

The processes "dis-ease or ease" are defined here as a field made up of environmental challenges, tissue responses, signs and symptoms, cognitive evaluations, global behaviors, and value-confirming life-styles (Fig. 1-2). Biogenesis enters the system, so to speak, primarily, but not exclusively, and becomes manifest with the elaboration of objectively discernible tissue responses/signs and

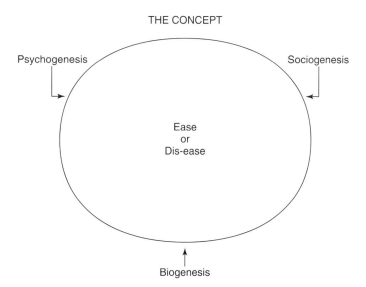

**Figure 1-1.**
The biopsychosocial concept.

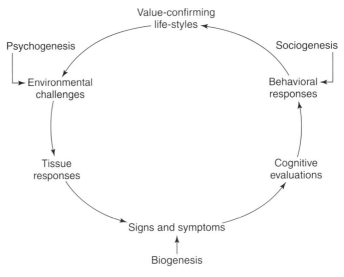

**Figure 1-2.**
The biopsychosocial approach to the process of disease or dis-ease.

symptoms. Sociogenesis enters the system and becomes manifest primarily by the elaboration of objectively discernible behaviors, whereas psychogenesis becomes manifest through objectively discernible environmental challenges. Cognitions, values, and sensations generated by tissue responses are subjectively experienced and reported to or inferred by the observer, and hence are not objective in the same sense. Consider a patient.

> Tom Jones, a 29-year-old man, experiences a scratchy throat, feels feverish, decides he is sick, and behaves accordingly, making an "emergency" appointment to see his physician (follow the arrows on Fig. 1-2). He wonders if it is "strep," and feels anxious with the thought because he thinks of his younger brother who had strep throat and then rheumatic fever, and lives with residual damage to his heart. He is quite certain he should be given an antibiotic. (Tom Jones' dis-eases seem to be pharyngitis, and an uncomplicated [nonneurotic] fear response; and his ease, a comfort in seeking assistance from his physician. In the center stands Tom Jones' brain as a transducer.)

A physician with an impoverished, linear, biogenic model of disease could very well come to the conclusion after his or her evaluation that the patient suffered from a pharyngitis secondary to a Coxsackie virus infection, that only supportive medical therapy was indicated, and that an antibiotic should not be prescribed. Management of the disease has been determined, but management of Tom Jones, the person, the patient, is not complete.

A variation of the model that is emphasized in this review speaks simultaneously to psychiatry *and* to behavioral medicine (Fig. 1-3). Here, particular attention is paid by the physician to the description (symptom) and the observation of a particular emotion (sign). Environmental challenge becomes stress, tissue response be-

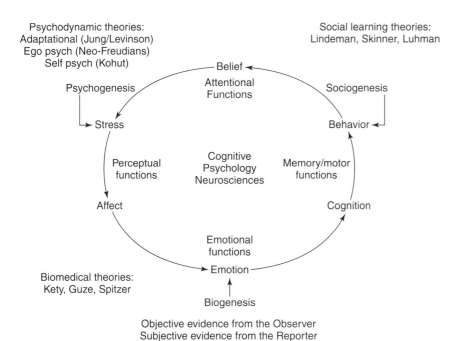

**Figure 1-3.**
Variation of the biopsychosocial model relative to psychiatry and behavioral medicine with integration of symptoms and emotions.

comes affect, and life-style becomes belief. This variation is particularly useful because the primary emotions seem to have a universality in facial display (signs), a common developmental history, and an increasingly understood neurophysiology.

A brief preview, by example, might be useful (see Fig. 1-3 and Table 1-1). Fear, whether biogenically or psychogenically induced,

**TABLE 1-1.**

## Biopsychosocial Model of Primary Emotions

| Stress | Affect | Emotion | Cognition | Behavior | Belief |
|--------|--------|---------|-----------|----------|--------|
| The familiar | Mastery | Acceptance | Known | Incorporative | Confidence Competence |
| The unexpected | Arousal | Surprise | New | Orienting | Exploration Examination |
| The noxious | Repulsion | Disgust | Alien | Rejecting | The vulgar (profane) |
| A gain | Gratification | Joy | Reward Pleasure | Reproducing | The sacred (valuable) |
| An injury | Anxiety | Fear | Danger | Avoidant Fleeting | Helplessness |
| A frustration | Aggression | Anger | Deprivation | Compulsive Assertive | Self and other control |
| A loss | Grief | Sadness | Abandonment | Dependent Withdrawing | Hopelessness |

tends to trigger in the subject the cognitive evaluation "danger," which in turn often becomes manifest to the observer in the subject's avoidant or fleeing behavioral responses. Sociogenic input has considerable influence in shaping this response. Many such behaviors over time result in a belief in one's basic helplessness in the world. An unrealistic (neurotic) sense of helplessness makes an individual in turn even more vulnerable to stresses that seem, or are injurious, and hence, a feedback loop, a cybernetic circuit, is created. A first and then a second version in the history of our patient:

> Tom Jones, in fact, grew up in a social environ that emphasized self-sufficiency. That, plus his experience with his little brother, resulted in a determination not to succumb to disease, to master his threatening world, to obtain an antibiotic.

Or,

> Tom Jones, in fact, grew up in a social environ that emphasized dependence on expert authorities. Hence, he "ran" to his doctor with the first sign of a "strep throat," wants to believe his doctor is right, but worries his diagnosis may be missed and he might repeat his brother's experience, perhaps deservedly.

Study Figure 1-3 and Table 1-1 for anger, sadness, and so forth.

This biopsychosocial model of disease might be seen as paradigmatic. A paradigm is a collection of concepts, theories, and ideas that delineate a given field. One might say that medicine, and its various disciplines, are preparadigmatic because a single paradigm has not emerged! Instead, medicine must attend to multiple systems, and systems with multiple levels of organization. Medicine, I suggest, is a polyparadigmatic science. Indeed, a particular theory of disease may be especially powerful in one situation but not another. "Power" refers to a theory's explanatory and predictive capability.

Within medicine generally, perhaps especially within psychiatry and behavioral medicine, there are competing theories (see Fig. 1-3). Some theories are more powerful in one context than another. Various psychodynamic theories are particularly powerful within the assumption of psychogenesis, but are not particularly useful given an assumption of biogenesis. Similar statements can be made for biomedical theories or social learning theories. For example, a learned helplessness theory of depression may be explanatory in understanding certain patients, but relatively impotent in working with patients with recurring unipolar depression. In this instance a biomedical theory usually has greater utility for the physician. This theory in turn loses power in the context of patients who experience recurring depressions secondary to losses to which they are particularly vulnerable. Disciples of a given theory often try to make their model all encompassing, but in stretching the theory, its power diminishes. Furthermore, its overapplication may tend to preserve a linear view of disease. The biopsychosocial model of disease, by contrast, attempts to bridge theories. It follows from a dialogue between the fields of cognitive psychology and neurobiology. It is polyparadigmatic. It requires more than one way of thinking.

Effective physicians diagnose disease. But they do not stop there; they diagnose the patient as well. It is not enough to engage in a disease-oriented clinical practice. Effective physicians integrate a patient-oriented and a population-based clinical practice as well (Fig. 1-4). Increasingly, national certifying examinations attempt to define minimum competence within the context of this integration. Increasingly, patient satisfaction and other outcome measures confront physicians, especially in mature managed care settings.

In summary, in the center of this field stands **disease**. From another perspective, in the center stands the **brain**. Operationally, and of particular import to a health professional, stands the **patient**.

## PSYCHIATRY AND BEHAVIORAL MEDICINE

Psychiatry is a science and a medical specialty. As a science, it seeks to understand disorders of the psyche (mind). The term "mind" is part of a psychological language reference system, along with such concepts as personality, anxiety, ego, and neurosis. The organ of the mind is the brain. The term "brain" is part of a physiologic language reference system, along with such concepts as neurotransmitters, the limbic system, and higher cortical functions. The

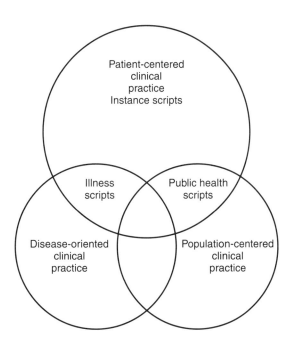

**Figure 1-4.**
Integration of disease-oriented, patient-oriented, and population-centered clinical practice.

process of the brain is the mind. Psychiatry uses both language systems. As a medical specialist, a psychiatrist seeks to study, diagnose, treat, and prevent mental, emotional, behavioral, and psychophysiological disorders, and adverse psychological responses to illness. Although these five areas of major concern overlap, most students of the field distinguish between them.

The term "behavioral medicine," as used here, denotes the practice by any physician of whatever specialty who consciously and deliberately diagnoses disease, in the classic sense, and the patient. Disease-oriented and patient-centered practice are thereby integrated. The function of the patient's brain is not divorced from the function of the patient's heart, or vice versa. In addition, population-based practice is increasingly necessary as health care systems move toward managed care models (see Fig. 1-4).

The mind, emotions, behavior, and soma (body) of a given patient are influenced by many factors—so many that it becomes difficult to define the limits of psychiatry and behavioral medicine. There are various language systems for describing human behavior, multiple theories to facilitate understanding, and even a variety of medical nomenclatures. No wonder the student may find this perplexing (all physicians are forever students). Nonetheless, despite these difficulties and differences, there is considerable agreement as to the major clinical entities and their management. Different patients with different personalities are understandable. Biogenesis, psychogenesis, and sociogenesis come together in the model previously described.

**Mental illness** is ubiquitous. Epidemiologic studies demonstrate that approximately 25% to 30% of visits to ambulatory care medical facilities can be attributed directly to mental illness. Most of these visits relate to the manifestations of anxiety and of depression. At any one time, as many patients with mental illnesses occupy hospital beds as do all other patients combined, even though the number of patients resident in state and county mental hospitals has decreased over the last several decades. In the United States, approximately 1 in 10 people will be hospitalized in a psychiatric hospital or a psychiatric unit during their lifetime. Many others are admitted to general hospitals. One person in every three or four will seek specific medical assistance for a mental disorder. Increasing numbers of patients are being seen in community mental health centers and hospital emergency rooms.

These figures and statements do not even include patients with **psychosomatic illnesses**, or those who present with adverse psychological responses to disease, and virtually every disease has accompanying psychological consequences. No wonder, then, that studies indicate that 75% to 90% of all patients present with psychological factors playing some role in their discomfiture. Add to this the increasingly recognized problem of compliance, that is, the relatively low percentage of patients who follow their prescribed medical regimen, and the mounting interest in prevention, and one can understand the current resurgence of interest in psychiatry and behavioral medicine. Undergraduate and graduate medical curricula have placed increased emphasis on neurobiology, behavioral sciences, psychiatry, and psychological or behavioral medicine. This, in turn, is reflected nationally on certification, licensure, and specialty examinations. New methodologies are testing knowledge, efficiency in data gathering, interpersonal skills, clinical judgment, effective management of disease, and effective management of patients. Computer-based simulations can even identify those physicians who tend to make dangerous management decisions.

Primary care physicians frequently work with patients who **somatize**, that is, focus on their body, tend to ignore or deny psychological dimensions to their illness, and resist efforts at psychological intervention. Less well recognized is another group of patients who **psychologize**, that is, tend to ignore their body or the possibility of illness in their body and resist appropriate biologic intervention. The physician by education, training, and role is potentially in a unique position to help both groups of patients.

Psychiatry in the United States has undergone a major change in its diagnostic nomenclature. The *Diagnostic and Statistical Manual of Mental Disorders* (*DSM-IV*) published by the American Psychiatric Association is officially in use. Therefore, the language and outline of *DSM-IV* are followed in this review. Where necessary, comparable terms are placed in parentheses so the reader can correlate this material with the various nosologies used by many texts still in print.

# Chapter 2

# Patient Evaluation

When evaluating patients and patient populations, certain critical concepts are essential to facilitate complete diagnoses and positive therapeutic outcomes. Of central significance is the biopsychosocial model already discussed. There are others; some are related to each other.

## Empirical Parallelism

Modern clinicians in their thinking and in their approach to patients avoid the historical mind/brain/body trichotomy still inherent in our language system. They function from the thesis of empirical parallelism. With any human event, there is the component that is experienced—for example, any phenomenal event of seeing, hearing, thinking, wishing, and feeling. The **subjective** experience of the event can be partially communicated to another with words, but only partially. The other component of the event is that observed by those others outside the event. When these observations are consensually validated, we tend to call the evidence **objective**. Examples are a neurophysiologic or neurochemical response in the brain or a behavior that accompanies such events. By the parallelism thesis, these two components, the subjective and objective, are not separate events, nor does one cause the other. A given thought does not cause a given neurophysiologic response, nor does the neurophysiologic event cause the thought. There is instead a single unitary event. In parallel, empirically, what I experience, you observe; what you experience, I observe. What each of us experience is subjective; what each of us observe can become objective.

This concept when applied to the clinical setting has practical consequences. Physicians should recognize that what the patient experiences is not necessarily what we see or hear. What we see, the patient may not experience. The question of whether the patient's problem is a physical illness or an emotional disturbance is usually a useless and often a deceptive, even dangerous dichotomy. *Only patients can experience their distress or declare their dis-ease*. It is not the physician's task to decide if someone is sick. The physician's task is to help the patient understand his or her dis-ease process, and given that understanding, help the patient with appropriate intervention. The mind/brain/body trichotomy can no longer be supported by the weight of scientific evidence. Physics has understood this for several decades. It is puzzling that biology and medicine have lagged so far behind. To hold this view, as unfortunately many physicians, including psychiatrists, still do, is to risk inefficiency, ineffectiveness, and even harm.

## Multiple Etiology

Any event (or constellation of events) labeled "disease" is multiply determined. The psychiatric term for this is "overdetermined." More often than not in medical practice, it is no longer useful to assume that for a given effect there is a given cause. Rather, we deal with multiple causality, multiple factors, and multiple determinants in any disease process. Hence, multiple interventions at multiple levels are usually required.

## Individual Versus Stimulus–Response Specificity

These two concepts originate in physiology, but their theoretic scientific underpinnings derive from the fields of chaos and quantum mechanics, respectively. **Individual response specificity** states that before one can predict the response of a given human to a given stimulus, one must first understand the individual. Or, given a particular response, one can reconstruct the events leading to that response only by knowing the individual organism. Only in the individual is there a specific response to a specific stimulus. More often than not, this applies to the practice of medicine with most patients most of the time.

The **stimulus–response specific assumption** states that a lawful, predictable relation exists between the stimulus and the response; therefore, one can predict the response simply by knowing the stimulus or reconstruct the stimulus by knowing the response. Knowledge about a particular, unique individual is not required. A light falling on the eye constricts the pupil. This assumption is very efficient and powerful when applicable. It has been and continues to be valuable in the development of scientific medicine. However, many physicians attempt to use this model, often unknowingly, when it simply does not apply.

Understanding and distinguishing between these two models and knowing when one is more applicable than the other is critical to the day-by-day, even moment-by-moment, practice of medicine. When used appropriately, these two complementary concepts shape the priorities of the doctor–patient interaction and enhance accuracy of evaluation and effectiveness of intervention. Upper airway obstruction is upper airway obstruction. Appropriate and effective intervention is nearly identical across patients. But a generalized anxiety disorder in one patient is not like the disorder in another. **Effective intervention** for one patient is different than for another. And the same applies for diabetes or appendicitis. Protocol medicine standardizes intervention of disease; if it is updated, as we learn more, it potentially enhances outcome. Unfortunately, protocols tend to ignore the individual, the uniquely dis-eased patient. If followed slavishly, as if the stimulus–response assumption always applied, as if the management of one personality is the same as for another, outcome deteriorates.

## The Major Threat to the Health of Man Is Man Himself

Health professionals of necessity must become interested in whatever threatens the life of their patients. Over time, the nature of this threat has changed and our understanding has changed as well. Hence, the focus of attention for one generation of physicians can never be exactly the same as for the next.

Clearly, the major source of change has derived, not from the threat from without, but the threat we pose to ourselves and each other by our behavior. There are numerous examples. The major cause of death in children younger than 5 years of age in the United States is now child abuse and child neglect. The major cause of death among medical students is suicide. For physicians, suicide occurs at approximately twice the rate of the general population. In the United States, in the 15- to 24-year-old category, the three leading causes of death are accidents, homicides, and suicide; they account for 75% of all deaths. Homicide rates for the United States, France, Britain, and Japan per 100,000 population are 10.2, 0.9, 1.0, and 1.3, respectively. In 1994, that meant 25,000 homicides in the United States. Why such a difference? The homicide rate for men in this age category in the United States is four times higher than in the next leading country for which statistics are available, Scotland. The United States has a greater percentage of its population in prison than any other developed country in the world.

Note the **leading causes of death** as recorded on death certificates on Table 2-1 and compare them with actual causes from a recent published study. A separate Institute of Medicine study concludes that 50% of the mortality of the 10 leading causes of death can be traced to life-styles. The Centers for Disease Control and Prevention publishes monthly an estimate of years of life lost in that cohort younger than 65 years of age. Accidents are now number one and account for 27% of the years lost. In fact, the years lost through accidents, homicides, and suicides exceed the years lost from cancer and heart disease!

Most knowledgeable health scholars hold that the single most significant factor affecting the health and life of people over the next 50 years is humanity's inability to date to control its birth rate. By mid-1994, our world population was 5.7 billion, double the population of 40 years ago. Over the past decade, food production has increased by 20%, but population has outstripped that so food pro-

**TABLE 2-1.**

**Leading Causes of Death in the United States, 1990 (2,148,000 deaths)**

| Death Certificates | | Actual Causes* | | |
|---|---|---|---|---|
| Cause | No. | Cause | No. | % |
| 1. Heart disease | 720,000 | 1. Tobacco | 400,000‡ | 19 |
| 2. Cancer | 505,000 | 2. Diet/activity | 300,000‡ | 14 |
| 3. Cerebrovascular disease | 144,000 | 3. Alcohol | 100,000‡ | 5 |
| 4. Accidents | 92,000 | 4. Microbes | 90,000 | 4 |
| 5. Chronic obstructive pulmonary disease | 87,000 | 5. Toxic agents | 60,000 | 3 |
| 6. Pneumonia and influenza | 80,000 | 6. Firearms | 35,000‡ | 2 |
| 7. Diabetes mellitus | 48,000 | 7. Sexual behavior | 30,000‡§ | 1 |
| 8. Suicide | 31,000† | 8. Motor vehicles | 25,000‡ | 1 |
| 9. Chronic liver disease | 26,000 | 9. Illicit drugs | 20,000‡ | <1 |
| 10. Human immunodeficiency virus infection | 25,000 | | | 50% |

**Other Factors Difficult to Quantify**

1. Lack of access to reliable primary care: 7% of premature deaths, 15% of potential years of life lost before age 65 years.

2. Poverty: in Canada, 11 fewer years of disability-free life despite guaranteed access to medical care.

3. National investment in prevention less than 5% of total annual health care cost.‖

*Data from JM McGinnis and WH Force, Actual Causes of Death in the United States, JAMA 1993; 270:2207.
†Estimated to be considerably higher than reported.
‡Predominant factor here is behavior.
§Includes human immunodeficiency virus, excess infant mortality with unintended pregnancy, hepatitis B, cervical cancer.
‖Data from Centers for Disease Control and Prevention.

duction per person has decreased by 10%. Fewer calories have been consumed per person in the world each successive year over the last 10 years. In a "Warning to Humanity," published in 1992, a document signed by well over a thousand world scientists, including over a hundred Noble Laureates, the conclusion is reached that currently we do not have a sustainable world society. We all live in a global village. The United States cannot build a wall around itself and keep itself isolated from the rest of the world. We do not have a sustainable society. Although many physicians are having difficulty confronting the reality, we currently do not have a sustainable health care system as well.

In summary, today the major threat to life and health does not come from the external environment, but from people themselves. The evidence is overwhelming: *the major challenge facing humankind is the creation of sustainable society.*

All this says that physicians of every discipline must become increasingly conversant with the anatomy of human behavior.

Prevention- and population-based clinical practice must receive increasing emphasis. Practicing cost-effective medicine is clearly a priority into the next century.

# PURPOSE OF THE INTERVIEWING–EVALUATING PROCESS

Although seemingly almost self-evident, it is useful, nonetheless, to keep in mind the various purposes of the interviewing–evaluating process. These may be outlined as follows:

1. To give patients the opportunity to **express** and **share** their **distress**. There is abundant evidence that this in itself diminishes the distress, facilitates the healing process, and enhances compliance.
2. To **observe** and to **elicit data**. Effective physicians see and hear with greater accuracy than those less effective. They even notice what they do not see and do not hear.
3. To **establish rapport**, or an effective working relationship. Patient satisfaction is linked to better outcomes. The positive attribute of physicians rated highest by their patients is that the physician "listens to me."
4. To develop **understanding of the disease** in question and the **patient with the disease**. Conscious, deliberate diagnosis of the patient, understanding the uniqueness of the patient, is frequently missing in patient encounters and leads to poorer outcome.
5. To **exchange information** with the patient. The second leading positive attribute of physicians as rated by patients is that they "explain things."
6. To develop a **working contract** and an **intervention strategy**, and to **effect implementation** of that strategy (see section on Characteristics of Effective Physicians, page 104).

# EVALUATION PROCESS

A prerequisite for an **effective evaluation process** is an understanding of the doctor–patient relationship and skill in developing that relationship. Another is knowing how to use certain communication styles when interviewing. A thorough knowledge of the phenomenology of mental processes is required, as is an understanding of the dynamics of human behavior. Perceptual accuracy must be honed. Given all of the above, interaction with a patient proceeds, it is hoped, toward a positive outcome.

With the **interrogative interview**, the patient is asked to follow and respond to the physician's associations. The technique is one primarily of asking a series of specific questions, in the hopes of obtaining a series of specific answers. Patients are invited to talk about their signs and symptoms. There is a deliberate effort to cut through so-called irrelevant information; hence the stereotypical questions of the review of systems. Historically, this approach tended to search for an etiology. The physician acted by doing something to the patient. However, information obtained solely through this interview process may have poor reliability and validity.

In contrast, in the **associative interview**, the physician follows and responds to the patient's associations. The patient is encouraged to talk about himself or herself, his or her life pattern, relationship with significant others, physical symptoms, and feeling responses. Again, the physician is obtaining information regarding symptoms and signs, but this time with a different technique. The physician is attempting to find out something about the organism, about the person who is ill, and not simply something about the illness itself. Irrelevant information tends to be what the health professional introduces. Here, the underlying assumption is one of multiple etiology or multiple factors in pathogenesis. Finally, the physician is more likely to act by working with the patient. The patient must participate. However, information obtained solely through this process may be incomplete; specific data needed by the physician may be missing.

Good interviews use a mixture of both techniques. In certain instances, one is more indicated than another.

## Interviewing Priorities

Usually the encounter begins with the patient and the physician confronting each other visually. Very early in the encounter, often with a glance, the physician determines whether there is an immediate medical emergency (e.g., major respiratory distress, cardiac arrest). Next, observing the **patient's behavior**, the clinician makes a fairly early and accurate judgment as to whether the patient is oriented, in contact with the surround. Evidence for the possibility of delirium or dementia would have a major influence on the nature of the remaining interaction. A skilled clinician can usually determine whether there may be a profound **thought disorder** by carefully listening to the content and the process of the patient's speech. In the overwhelming number of instances, there is no immediate medical emergency, and the patient is oriented and does not demonstrate a thought disorder of psychotic proportions. In short, the physician has another "brain" with which to work.

Next should come the question, "What is it that I would like to know next?" From the principle of individual response specificity, comes the answer, "I would like to know something fairly reliable about the nature of this particular individual at this moment in time." The answer to the question is *not* the chief complaint; that will come soon enough. "Understanding the patient tells me how to proceed." The royal road to understanding a given individual at a given moment is to conduct an inventory of that individual's primary emotions. The answer is another question, "What is this patient's primary emotion?"

## Identifying the Primary Emotions and Obtaining Congruence

Let us take a specific example. A male family physician in an office setting introduces himself to his next patient and notes that she is in no acute medical distress and seems oriented. This is not a medical emergency. She is breathing satisfactorily, her heart is beating, there is no evidence of shock, and her brain is functioning effectively. She appears to be in her mid-30s, is neatly and well dressed, is sitting on the edge of her chair with one foot ahead of the other, and greets him with wide open eyes. She licks her lips and says at the height of inspiration, "I'm certainly glad to see you." Many physicians in this situation would then say something like, "Thank you. Well, what brings you to see me?" But a more efficient and a more effective response is something on the order of, "Thank you. Do you feel a bit anxious?" With this, the patient responds, "Frankly, Doctor, I'm more than anxious. I'm scared to death. A week ago, while riding my horse, I hit my head on the limb of a tree. I felt a little dazed but not anything else and I went on with the ride, but several days later I started having headaches unlike any kind of headaches I've ever had in my life and I'm worried that maybe I have a subdural hematoma like my younger sister had after an automobile accident."

This patient looks anxious or fearful. The physician wonders if she feels anxious. He structures his response accordingly. Indeed, through her words, it is clear: she feels anxious and fearful. The objective and subjective evidence, the behavioral and the verbal evidence, are **congruent**. Psychologically healthy people in trusting situations "look how they feel and feel how they look." (The price a person pays for looking a feeling but not feeling it is forever being puzzled why other people respond to them the way they do. The price a person pays who feels a feeling and says so but does not look it is the price of forever not being believed.) When patients are congruent, they generally have a very good idea why they are feeling the way they are feeling. If this information is not volunteered, the physician can ask and the answer usually can be taken at face value. This particular patient volunteers this information in a direct and succinct manner.

The first step, then, in an interview process, is to ask oneself questions about the patient's **primary emotion**. Do I **hear words** indicating that the patient is aware of this emotion? Do I **see evidence** that portrays this emotion? In short, is the patient congruent? If the patient presents objective evidence of anger, for example, the clinician must determine whether the patient is aware of feeling angry. If not, the patient is incongruent. If the patient states that he or she is feeling a particular way in the absence of objective evidence for that particular emotional state, the effective interviewer notes that discrepancy and often draws the patient's attention to that incongruity. Patients with neurotic conflict tend to be incongruent in one fashion or another. Patients' words and behaviors often suggest the particular **defense mechanisms** whereby they either hide their feelings from others or hide their feelings from themselves. Further, such patients usually are not completely aware of the factors that precipitate the feeling as experienced or portrayed. They are more difficult patients. However, this was not the case with our example.

### *Primary Emotions*

When the **face** expresses a primary emotion in an undisguised fashion, it is universal and independent of culture, race, sex, or age. Each primary emotion has an understood and distinct neurophysiology. Each emotion is accompanied by a typical body response. Each emotion is considerably shaped or modified by experience. Each person has been trained to express, show, hide, or disguise such responses. Each is trained to see or not to see such evidence in another.

Perception is not veridical; it is a construction. Students can come to medical school, graduate, become physicians, and practice medicine for a lifetime without discovering what it is they do not see. To see accurately requires a particularly effective learning experience.

Research has amply demonstrated that many physicians simply do not see the evidence. Do not assume that you do. You did not come to medical school having been trained not to feel an enlarged liver. But we do come having been trained not to notice or respond to the objective or subjective evidence of certain emotions. An unlearning process is necessary before learning can even begin. If I do not see evidence of depression, even though I know what the criteria for a diagnosis of depression may be, I do not make the diagnosis. Hence, I do not treat it. In study after study, therefore, physicians of both sexes underdiagnose depression, especially in men, and overdiagnose anxiety in women. Obviously such physicians have poorer outcomes. The problem is that when we do not see something, for example, objective evidence for anxiety in a man, we do not even know that we do not see it!

The **primary emotions** are:

1. Acceptance, comfort
2. Disgust
3. Surprise
4. Joy
5. Fear, anxiety
6. Anger
7. Sadness

These emotions are listed in the order in which they appear developmentally. Infants respond to faces portraying these emotions differentially and before they respond to words. There is a greater volume of our brain devoted to recognizing faces than to recognizing words. Throughout life, nonverbal behavior usually is a more powerful evocator of response in the other than verbal behavior.

Study the photographs on this page. Ask yourself, what are these faces saying? Commit yourself to an answer. Then refer to the appendix at the end of the text and to the questions and discussion. In

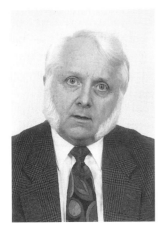
**Photograph 1**

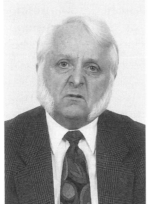
**Photograph 2**

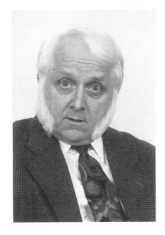
**Photograph 3**

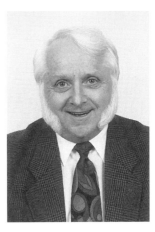
**Photograph 4**

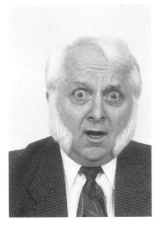
**Photograph 5**

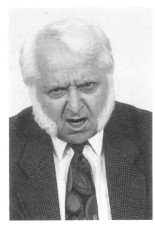
**Photograph 6**

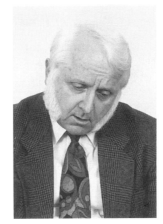
**Photograph 7**

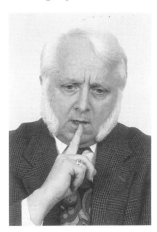
**Photograph 8**

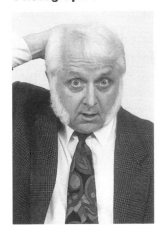
**Photograph 9**

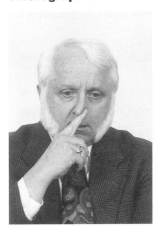
**Photograph 10**

the process, you may gain some insight into what you tend not to see or tend to mislabel.

Other emotions are secondary and are derivative from the primary. They are not expressed facially or nonverbally in a universal manner.

The most common face of patients when seen by their physician in an outpatient setting is comfort. Most patients who know their physicians are comfortable with them. The second is joy; they are pleased to see them. Working with these patients is relatively easy. It is patients who are dis-eased, who present with objective evidence of disgust, fear, anger, or sadness, or some combination, who may be difficult. Objective evidence refers to behavior. Nonverbal communication is nonpropositional (not as likely to be false), spontaneous, and biologically structured.

Subjective evidence refers to words. Verbal communication is propositional, intentional, and culturally structured. I cannot really know how someone feels unless he or she tells me. When a patient says "I feel nervous," ordinarily the physician can assume that the patient is experiencing distress, but the physician does not know if "nervous" means frightened, (i.e., fear, anxiety) or if it means a sense of muscle tension accompanying anger, frustration, or the like.

### Primer of Emotions

Emotional states and reactions are viewed as reflections of underlying **affective disturbances** triggered by **stresses** and, hence, should be of considerable interest to the physician.

#### SUBJECTIVE EVIDENCE
Subjective evidence refers to the patient's verbal description of the experienced emotion. The emotion experienced and then shared through words allows a person partially to know the other's experience. Categories 1 through 6 may suggest some level of subjective awareness, but in decreasing order. Categories 7 and 8 are *not* evidence for conscious awareness, but should alert the listener to look very carefully for nonverbal evidence to the contrary (i.e., incongruence between subjective and objective evidence).

1.  "I am" statements. Patients may use a term suggesting a less intense emotion than they actually feel, or the intense feeling may be dampened by a variety of mechanisms, hence, for example, "timid" rather than "terrified" (Table 2-2).
2.  "I feel like" statements. Patients may be unable or unwilling to describe *how* they feel in terms as outlined above, but instead, describe what they feel like doing. This suggests some level of awareness, although not to the degree of statements under category 1 (Table 2-3).
3.  Statements that compare present feeling to a past feeling under certain circumstances (e.g., "I feel like I did when I had my tonsils out").

**TABLE 2-2.**

**Terms Used in "I Am" Statements**

| Fear | Anger | Sadness | Disgust |
|---|---|---|---|
| Timid, shy, apprehensive, nervous, anxious, frightened, fearful, panicked, scared, terrified | Disinterested, annoyed, irritated, mad, angry, hateful, furious | Pensive, wistful, gloomy, sad, dejected, sorrowful, depressed, grief-stricken | Tired, bored, dislike, disgusted, nauseated, loathing, scornful |

4. Statements that directly describe physiologic reactions or concomitants (see next section, "Objective Evidence").
5. Figures of speech—may be linked to an emotional state. These often derive from accompanying physiologic responses (Table 2-4).
6. Statements that suggest secondary emotions, and hence, to a degree mask a primary emotion. Secondary emotions are learned, often, at least in part, by combining several primary emotions. Table 2-5 is a guide to the subject. What is significant clinically is to recognize the primary emotion "buried" in these other terms.
7. Statements that repeatedly or too emphatically deny an emotion when this is unlikely (e.g., "I've never been angry in my life").
8. At times the patient may substitute one emotion for another, usually a positive one for a negative one, and this may be reflected in his or her verbal description (e.g., "I enjoy his company. He is so intelligent, but . . . well, no, he is really a fine person").

**OBJECTIVE EVIDENCE**

Objective evidence refers to the examiner's observations. These observations may or may not correlate with the patient's verbal description (i.e., there may or may not be congruence).

**TABLE 2-3.**

**Actions Described in "I Feel Like" Statements**

| Fear | Anger | Sadness | Disgust |
|---|---|---|---|
| Running, hiding, screaming, shaking, trembling inside, crying, laughing, falling apart | Hitting, bashing in the wall, killing, knocking his block off, slamming the door, shouting | Crying, giving up, going away, going to bed, dying, empty | Turning away, running away, vomiting, hiding |

---
**TABLE 2-4.**

**Figures of Speech**

| Fear | Anger | Grief or Sorrow | Disgust |
|------|-------|-----------------|---------|
| Cold feet, cold sweat, shaking in boots, scared to death, petrified, hair stood on end, knees knocking, blood turned to ice, white as a ghost, butterflies in stomach, shit (or pissed) my pants, lost my marbles | Hot under the collar, in a sweat, livid, saw red, gnashing teeth, steaming, bristling with rage, fighting mad, hopping mad, got my goat, pissed me off, pain in the neck, pain in the ass, shove it, shit on it, fuck it | Cry inside, giving up the ghost, what's the use, why keep trying, lost soul, I have nothing left, that's the way the cookie crumbles | Makes me sick, gives me the creeps, slimy, it smells, it stinks, piss on it, shit on it |

---

1. Facial expressions—refer to Table 2-6 for a tentative outline and guide. Facial expressions are the most accurate and reliable indicators of a given emotion.
2. Body attitude, gestures, and so on (Table 2-7)
3. Speech characteristics (see Table 2-7)
4. Physiologic responses (see Table 2-7)

Obviously, this section is far from complete. Readers are encouraged to add observations of their own. There are two notes of caution, however. First, all patients do not express or display their fear or anger in exactly the same way. Second, many patients express and display a mixture of emotions (e.g., fear and anger, anger and sadness). Each patient must be assessed individually.

---
**TABLE 2-5.**

**Secondary Emotions Resulting from Combinations of Primary Emotions**

|  | Fear | Anger | Sadness | Disgust | Joy |
|--|------|-------|---------|---------|-----|
| **Joy** | Guilt | Pride, confidence, revenge | Sentimentality | Morbidness | |
| **Surprise** | Awe, alarm, apprehension, dread | Outrage | Disappointment | Horror, distrust, embarrassment | Delight |
| **Acceptance** | Submission | Dominance, revenge, resentment, stubbornness | Resignation, sentimentality, pessimism | Cynicism, shame | Optimism |
| **Sadness** | Guilt, despair | Envy, jealousy, sullenness | | Misery, remorse | |
| **Disgust** | Shame, embarrassment, prudishness | Scorn, contempt | Misery, remorse | | |
| **Anger** | Guilt | | | | |

**TABLE 2-6.**

**Facial Expressions as Indicators of Emotion**

|  | Fear | Anger | Sadness | Disgust |
|---|---|---|---|---|
| Eyebrows | Raised | Frowning, knit | Flat | Some frowning |
| Eyelids | Wide open | Tensely narrowed | Half closed | Occasional squint |
| Eyes | Pupils dilated, fixed stare | Pupils constricted, glare | Red, tears, downcast | Turning away |
| Mouth | Open, round or rectangular, trembling of lips, dry mouth, licking of lips | Open, elliptical, tense grin, lips retracted or compressed, teeth clenched | Inverted crescent, relaxed | At times movements suggesting vomiting, sneer, protruding lower lip, prominent nasolabial folds |
| Face | White, "cold" sweat | Red, veins distended, masseters prominent, nostrils widened | Pale, lengthened muscles, flaccid | Nostrils raised |
| Head | Fixed, pulling away | Toward object, jutting jaw | Hanging | Turning away |
| Respiration | Inspiratory tendency, yawning | Expiratory tendency | Sighing, slow and feeble | Tendency to hold breath |

## EVIDENCE OF PHYSICIAN RESPONSE TENDENCIES

A third class of evidence pertains to the **professional's awareness of his or her own response tendencies** to certain patients and their expressions of emotion. Each professional must determine this for himself. For example, one physician may have a tendency to "rush in and rescue" depressed patients, another may have a tendency to get angry, and another may become sad.

**TABLE 2-7.**

**Body Attitudes and Speech Characteristics Associated with Emotions**

|  | Fear | Anger | Sadness | Disgust |
|---|---|---|---|---|
| **Body Attitude** | "Flight," trembling, guarding gestures and posture, shifting, trivial hand occupation | "Attack"—tense muscles, fist clenched, quick, forceful gestures | Limp, helpless, few gestures, head shaking, hand wringing | Turning away and pushing away gestures, respiratory avoidance response |
| **Speech Characteristics** | Trembling, pauses, hesitates, blocking or rapid and disjointed; height of inspiration | Very controlled, precise, or forceful, loud, and the like; during expiration and controlled | Sighing, slow pace, retardation, end of expiration | Sneering quality, "snorting," sniffing, clearing of throat |

As a note of interest, consider Sir Arthur Conan Doyle, who was a physician. His creation, Sherlock Holmes, was modeled after Dr. Joseph Bell, a member of the medical school faculty at the University of Edinburgh. Doyle, his student, was greatly impressed by Bell's capacity for making accurate observations and then coming to amazingly accurate deductions. In a sense, the competent practitioner of psychological medicine is a kind of Sherlock Holmes.

## CLASSIFICATION OF NONVERBAL BEHAVIORS

**Expressors** are culture free and universal when expressed by the face in an undisguised fashion. They portray the primary emotions. They are subcortical in origin and extrapyramidal in motor expression. All the nonverbal behaviors that follow are culturally dependent, learned, cortical in origin, and pyramidal in motor expression. When the face expresses more than one emotion at a time, it is termed a blend. Sequences of emotions may appear rapidly.

**Illustrators** are behaviors that accompany verbal sentences and, as the term indicates, literally illustrate what is being said, most frequently with the hands.

**Regulators** are behaviors that serve to control the ebb and flow of communication. In our dominant culture, listening is indicated by looking at the person talking. If the person to whom we are talking does not look at us, we tend to believe they are not listening. However, there are cultures where this is not the case, and listening is indicated by not looking at the speaker. This is true, for example, among the Native American plains tribes. In our dominant culture, when talking, people may look to the left or to the right while collecting their thoughts, and looking away means that they are not through speaking. The skilled listener waits. The indicator of being through is when the speaker's eyes rest on listeners, accompanied, perhaps, by a drop in voice and a gentle nod of the head.

**Emblems** are nonverbal behaviors, often facial, that have a specific meaning all their own. For example, the upper half of the face of anger, but with a relaxed mouth, often with a finger to the lip, indicates "I'm thinking." The eyebrow and forehead of surprise in the absence of evidence in the eyes and mouth indicate "I'm asking you a question." In this instance, the person is not feeling surprised.

**Simulators** are nonverbal behaviors taught by society either to exaggerate or hide a primary emotion. One example is the so-called phony smile—namely, a smile of the lower half of the face. When the mouth is smiling, look to see if the eyes are smiling. If the eyes are not smiling, it is not joy. Another is the tight, thin lip, the phony face of acceptance. When the face looks blank, and seems comfortable and accepting, look at the mouth. If the mouth is tense, the emotion is not acceptance.

**Adaptors** are culture dependent to some degree, family dependent to a greater degree, and are particularly characteristic of a given individual, especially when under stress. The behavior is one that suggests how the person tends to adapt to a dis-easing emotion. Body posture, turn of the head, and the position and movements of hands and arms, as well as feet, suggest adaptors. The value in observing adaptors can be exemplified as follows.

Assume a surgeon is making rounds early in the morning, visiting in sequence three older men each of whom will have the same surgical procedure. The surgeon asks each one, "Are you all set for your surgery?" In each case, the patient's verbal response is, "Certainly." The first patient accompanies his response with a face of fear followed by a grooming gesture to the back of his head by his right hand. In the second, the face of fear is followed by a clearing of the throat, a sniffing, a rubbing of the base of the nose with the right forefinger (the respiratory avoidance response), and then a scratching of the cheek with the right hand. This might be called a nonverbal sentence.

Finally, in the last room, the face of fear is followed by a series of organizing gestures, checking to make sure that the upper button of his pajamas is buttoned, adjusting the sheets, finally bringing the hands together fingertip to fingertip (tenting). Given the evidence, which patient primarily needs reassurance from the physician? Which patient needs a detailed description of what will transpire before and immediately after surgery? Which patient is most likely to deny his discomfort, perhaps even the most prone to depression during the postoperative period? Managing anxiety appropriately before surgery has been shown to influence postoperative morbidity.

## Establishing Consensus Regarding the Stress

Once congruence is established, the patient and the physician usually can come to an agreement as to what may account for the distress fairly quickly. However, this may not be the case with many patients. They have been trained or have trained themselves not to show their distress or even be aware of it. Usually, this is accomplished through the elaboration of a neurotic personality. Accompanying this structure is often a lack of accurate awareness of the constellations of events, past and present, leading to the disease in question. In contrast, the patient in our example (page 17), a **genital character** (psychologically healthy, nonneurotic), looks anxious, feels anxious, knows why she is anxious, and is ready to work toward a solution with her physician. The physician's response might be, "Your anxiety is understandable. From what you have told me so far, a subdural hematoma, while possible, is unlikely." Consensus is established. There is agreement that feeling anxious and looking anxious, given the possibility of a subdural hematoma, makes sense. The diagnosis of the dis-ease is a normal fear reaction.

Effective physician interviewers tend verbally to summarize their understanding of the patient's visit before proceeding to the next step, making a contract. (Please note that this summary is not yet a summary of the present illness, but is usually more than a restatement of the chief complaint!)

Again, most patients seen in an ambulatory setting are known to the physician. Many show no evidence of a diseasing emotion. After greeting such a patient, the physician might say, "Well, how are you today?" The patient responds, "Fine." Noting evidence of comfort, that the patient indeed looks fine, the follow-up question might be "What brings you to see me?" In other words, with congruence for comfort or acceptance, with no signal indicating distress, the physician proceeds to the contract, following the therapeutic sequence (see Fig. 2-1).

But for patients who look or feel distressed, or both, the stress may not be so easily identifiable. Especially with nonneurotic patients (genital characters), there are expected linkages. With the emotion **fear**, ordinarily one expects the stress of **injury** or threat of injury, physical or psychological, in fact or in fantasy (e.g., the possibility of a subdural hematoma in our example). With **sadness**, one expects the stress of **loss**, real or symbolic, in fact or in fantasy. Anger is usually triggered by **frustration** of need (see Table 1-1 and review the expected sequence in the biopsychosocial model).

When the word arrives developmentally, so does culture, and culture has something to teach the developing child. Culture, families, and experience teach us **elicitor rules**—what it is that is supposed to elicit disgust, joy, fear, anger, or sadness. These rules are not the same for all patients, nor for all physicians. Culture teaches **display rules**—what emotions may be displayed and to whom and when. Here, there is a striking sexual double standard. Boys and men are taught not to show fear, not to cry; hence, a face of anger or a phony face of acceptance may hide an underlying sadness or fear. Girls and women are taught not to show anger, so they may cry instead, that is, they cry when angry. In other words, it's as neurotic for men to shout when scared as it is for women to cry when angry. In both instances these responses confuse the other—including the physician. Such "deceit" toward others, in time, can become a "deceit" toward self. Then, the precise nature of the stress triggering the dis-ease displayed or experienced may not be known at all, or at least imperfectly or incompletely known. When asked, "What's bothering you?" or "How do you understand your anxiety?" such a person may simply say he or she does not know, or utter an incomplete sentence. Helping such patients talk in complete sentences brings understanding and identifies the stress for both parties, the patient and the physician.

To help patients talk in complete sentences, physicians must first overcome their own **recognition rules**. Again, this requires an effective learning experience, one that is missing in most medical schools and in most residencies. Such rules are taught by our culture, our families, our experience, and our mentors. Perception is a construction, a matter of what I believe I will see or not see, hear or not hear. What is it I am not to see, not to hear, not to notice? What is it I am simply to assume? That is something each person must discover for himself or herself.

## Making a Contract

At this point in the process, effective physicians usually obtain the patient's **chief expectation**. In our continuing example, the physician might say, "I take it you're here to get to the bottom of these different kind of headaches you're having." The patient nods and says, "Yes, indeed!" What follows is an explicitly stated understanding of how the two of them will work together to solve the problem, including perhaps what length of time will be required for more detailed history taking, a physical examination, the possibility of gathering additional information, and a decision is reached and an agreement is made as to the nature of the problem. This sets the stage for the final step in the process of a therapeutic interaction.

## Developing a Strategy for Intervention and Implementation

The physician's particular knowledge of disease processes is very helpful to the patient. The patient's special knowledge of himself or herself, in turn, can be very helpful to the physician. Together they develop a strategy for intervention and create a specific plan for implementation. Each, then, proceeds to fill his or her particular role in that plan.

Again, national competency examinations are paying increased attention to the **measurement of interpersonal skills**. By attending to the steps outlined previously (see page 17), a candidate may answer a whole series of questions on such examinations. (See examples at the end of this chapter.) More important, patient outcome research increasingly points to the effectiveness of this particular sequence of enhancing therapeutic outcome. Training and practice are required for any physician to become an accurate diagnostician and an effective therapist, especially when the physician is working with the many patients who resist the process. I call this process the **therapeutic sequence** (Fig. 2-1). This process in some form is a

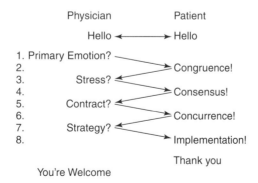

**Figure 2-1.**
The therapeutic sequence.

characteristic of more effective physicians of whatever discipline. (Again, effective means those whose patients have more positive outcomes.)

# STRUCTURE OF THE INTERVIEWING PROCESS

In the context of the **doctor–patient interaction** and during the process of **effective interviewing** as outlined previously, the clinician keeps in mind an historical outline. During and after the interview, the physician organizes this history into a particular format. In the practice of psychiatry and behavioral medicine, the structural outline of a usual medical history is perfectly appropriate and is not detailed here. The presenting complaint is significant and usually easily obtained, but again, for effective interviewers, it is not their first concern. In the preceding example, if the physician's first response or inquiry was toward the chief complaint, the patient would undoubtedly have presented her headaches. Typically, what would follow would be a series of questions and answers regarding the specific nature of the headaches. By paying attention first to the patient's emotional state, the physician elicited very salient information, after which can come the necessary medical interrogative interview and, in *less* time and with *greater* accuracy and with *better* outcome, information regarding the present illness and the past personal and family medical history.

Especially when psychological factors seem particularly significant to the patient's problem or to the doctor–patient interaction, it is frequently helpful, even necessary, to obtain a more detailed personal, familial, and social history. Special attention might be paid to growth and development issues, a history of present and past family relationships, an education and work history, and a history of leisure activities. Patients' descriptions of themselves as individuals and their descriptions of their significant others as personalities are often of special value. "What was your mother like as a person?" might be a typical question in this setting.

## Mental Status Examination

Also in the context of the interview process, a **mental status examination** is conducted. It is, if you will, a part of the physical examination, an examination of higher brain functions. Various authors arrange the content of the examination somewhat differently. The following outline is presented because meaningful diagnostic implications can be drawn from dysfunction reflected in the various groupings.

1. Sensorium
   *Consciousness:* level and stability
   *Orientation:* four spheres of person, time, place, and situation
   *Memory:* immediate, recent, and remote
   *Attention and concentration*
   > The first letters of these variables spell the *mnemonic* COMA, which is particularly meaningful because dysfunction in any of these four areas should alert the physician to a possible "organic" condition (i.e., delirium or dementia).
2. Thought process
   Production rate
   Continuity
   > Dysfunctions of thought process have implications for major psychotic-proportion affective and thought disorders, as well as delirium and dementia.
3. Thought content
   Relation to reality
   Concept formation: relative abstractability
   Intelligence
   Insight and judgment
   Characteristic topics
   > These parameters are disrupted mostly in the major thought disorders, but also in affective psychotic conditions. Certain topics of concern are common to the various personality disorders.
4. Perceptions
   Hallucinations
   Illusions
   > Dysfunction in perception should always alert the physician to possible delirium or dementia, as well as a major thought disorder.
5. Emotional regulation
   Subjective and objective evidence for emotional states and relative congruence
   Ambivalence
   Appropriateness to thought content
   > Disruptions here can accompany any major psychotic condition, especially thought disorders, but most commonly the problem lies within the realm of anxiety or depression spectrum disorders. Again, certain patterns are common to the various personality disorders.
6. Relevant somatic functioning
   Sleep
   Appetite
   Weight
   Sexual functioning
   > These are sometimes called vegetative behaviors. When dysfunctional in a syndrome complex, they suggest an accompanying affective disorder.

Some aspect of the traditional physical examination is required for evaluation purposes in most, but not all, instances in a medical setting. Indeed, on many occasions a rather thorough physical examination is in order even if the patient presents primarily with what seems like an emotional or mental problem. This is particularly true if the clinician suspects an organic mental disorder or a psychosomatic illness. In some patients, certain illnesses mimic a conversion disorder, just as conversion disorders often mimic certain physical conditions.

To diagnose the patient as a person always requires a "physical examination"; a given personality after all is a characteristic pattern of brain function. This examination, however, is conducted without a stethoscope; it is conducted with eyes and ears in the course of the therapeutic sequence, during the data gathering of a history, and during a formally conducted mental status examination, if this is indicated.

# EVALUATION BEYOND HISTORY, MENTAL STATUS, AND PHYSICAL EXAMINATION

## Involvement of Family, Friends, and Other Health Professionals

Perhaps next in significance to the evaluation of the patient is interviewing one or more members of the patient's family or friends. Their view of the problem can be extraordinarily valuable; their involvement with strategies for intervention may be crucial. This is especially true for children.

A review of the patient's past medical records is also too frequently overlooked, as is direct contact with other health professionals with whom the patient has worked.

## Psychological Tests

In some instances, **formal psychological testing** is helpful. Increasingly, and in ambulatory settings especially, various standardized scales for anxiety and depression are used. Standardized neuropsychological tests are especially helpful in diagnosing mental retardation, severe thought disorders, dementia, or specific deficits of cortical functions secondary to a variety of physical conditions.

## Laboratory Tests

When certain nosologic entities are suspected, specific imaging studies or laboratory tests are often indicated. These are covered under the various headings in the section on Nosology.

# Electroencephalographic Examination (EEG)

The EEG is a recording of the electrical activity of the brain. Leads are attached to the scalp, and the brain waves are recorded. The amplitude of normal brain activity is from 20 to 70 μV. Brain waves vary from 1 to 50 cycles/second. The most conspicuous activity is **alpha** waves, 8 through 13 cycles/second, especially seen in recordings from the occipital region. This rhythm tends to disappear when the eyes are opened, or when the subject is tense, engaged in mental activity, or experiencing considerable anxiety. In the normal waking population, **theta** activity is also seen, ranging from 4 to 7 cycles/second. **Delta** activity refers to waves under 4 cycles/second. Delta activity is very unusual in a normal waking person. When seen, it suggests sleep, delirium, or diffuse brain damage. When slow-wave activity seems to be localized over one area of the brain, it may suggest a space-occupying lesion. Fast activity beyond 13 cycles/second is called **beta** activity. Sudden bursts of high-voltage, disordered activity of a paroxysmal nature, different from background rhythm, are frequently seen in patients with a convulsive disorder. Random activity from recordings over the temporal lobe is reported with increased frequency in patients with temporal lobe epilepsy, but many patients without any lesion whatsoever also show occasional spiking in these areas. Some patients with temporal lobe epilepsy have normal EEGs. A characteristic pattern is often seen with petit mal epilepsy, namely, a pattern of 3 cycles/second spike and wave activity (spike and dome pattern).

It is often stated that the EEG is not of particular value in psychiatry. Although this may be true generally with the traditional recording techniques, sophisticated measurements involving computer analysis are making it clear that certain psychiatric illnesses are accompanied by dysrhythmias of one kind or another. Most of this work is still experimental and does not as yet have wide diagnostic or therapeutic application.

In the clinical setting, the EEG is useful primarily when a convulsive disorder of one kind or another is being considered, when a sleep study is indicated, or when the possibility of brain death is being evaluated.

# Imaging Studies

Of increasing significance in psychiatry are the various imaging technologies—that is, **computed tomography**, **magnetic resonance imaging**, and **positron emission tomography** scans. Given signs and symptoms of a **focal deficit** or a **space-occupying lesion**, they are of considerable value. Whether they will become useful for other domains of psychiatry and behavioral medicine in making diagnoses or in planning or in following treatment is still an open question. However, these studies already are contributing significantly to our understanding of brain function.

# THE THERAPEUTIC SEQUENCE IN ACTION: AN EXAMPLE

A family physician practicing for 10 years in a town, population 5000, is about to see a patient already known to him from previous visits. The patient is 55 years old, white, female, married for 33 years, and has three children, ages 26, 28, and 30 years. She is the manager of a small accounting firm and has previously been in good health, physiologically and psychologically. The patient walks into the consulting room and takes a seat. The physician shuts the office door.

PT: Good morning, Doctor John.

DR: Good morning Joan, you look worried. [The physician has noted the characteristic facies of moderate anxiety and a fidgeting quality in the patient's hand movements as she sits down. He chooses to use the more general term, "worried," in his first statement.]

PT: Yes. To tell you the truth, I'm scared. [The patient acknowledges the physician's perceptual accuracy and specifies more precisely her emotional state.]

DR: Scared about what, Joan? [The physician notes congruence between the emotion communicated and the emotion experienced, speculates that this person has experienced a recent stress of injury or threat of injury, and proceeds to obtain consensus.]

PT: Well, to be honest, I am scared that I may have heart trouble. You remember my dad had a heart attack several years ago, and it runs in the family. When I walk from my home to my office, you know, up that hill, for the last several weeks I've noticed this discomfort, this pain in my chest, and it kind of goes down my left arm . . . a classic description, I guess. I tried to pass it off at first, but it's happened now three or four times, especially if I'm hurrying, but I haven't noticed anything else. [Pauses, takes a deep breath.] But, I can't help thinking it might be some kind of heart trouble.

DR: So you're scared you might have heart trouble. That certainly would be something to be concerned about. It has run in your family, and what you've noticed is this pain in your chest and left arm when you are walking in a hurry up this hill to your office. Is that right? [The physician already has achieved a degree of consensus, is making sure the message sent has been the message received, is being appropriately nurturing, and accepts the patient's anxiety. In addition, he has introduced a modifying influence by the use of the word "concerned," and is ready to establish an appropriate contract.]

PT: Yes, that says it nicely.

DR: So in coming to see me, you want me to check this out?

PT: I sure do.

DR: OK. Well, I need to get a little more history, then I will want to examine you, and we may need to run some tests. We'll talk more about that later. Is that about what you expected?

PT: It certainly is. [Since both the physician and the patient have a clear understanding of what each expects, at this point there is concurrence.]
DR: Anything else?
PT: No.

The physician proceeds with the history, confirms the absence of other symptoms, confirms the accuracy of the patient's description of the pain, and based on the information seriously considers the diagnosis of coronary artery disease with angina pectoris. He determines that the patient has already discussed these symptoms with her husband, and he is also "very concerned." He then performs the appropriate physical examination, obtains a chest radiograph and ECG during this first office visit, and orders the appropriate laboratory studies. He sits down with the patient, reviews the evidence, shares his tentative diagnosis, and outlines a suggested diagnostic plan and a plan for therapeutic intervention. The patient agrees.

DR: Are there any questions or concerns? [The physician is looking for possible difficulties with implementation.]
PT: No, I guess not. [The patient licks her lips, and an anxious facial expression returns. The therapeutic sequence will be repeated.]
DR: Joan, you still seem rather concerned about something. What is it? [The physician hears the distortion and sees the anxiety and approaches it directly.]
PT: Doctor, I don't want to die.
DR: You're worried that somehow this means you're going to die?
PT: Well, I think you can understand that, given my family history.
DR: Yes, I certainly can. But, you have done several things that make a lot of sense. These symptoms have been present for only a few weeks. You haven't ignored them. You have come to see me. We are going to look at this very carefully before we jump to any conclusions. Even if this turns out to be what we both expect, we have some reason to be optimistic. There are things you can do, things I can do, things we can do. With appropriate treatment, we can anticipate fair success in managing the problem. [The physician continues to set the stage for shared responsibility and joint participation in the development of a therapeutic strategy and its implementation.]
PT: Yes, I know, but it is going to take me a while to get used to all of this.
DR: Yes, it will.
PT: And my husband is really worried.
DR: What would you think about your husband coming in with you next time? [The physician does not say, "I think your husband should come in next time."]
PT: I think that's a good idea. Well, I'll go ahead and get those tests and keep track of any other pains like we talked about. I understand about using the medicine, and my husband and I will come to see you in two days when we have the results of the tests. OK?

DR: Sounds good.
PT: OK, see you then. [Both stand up.] Thank you.
DR: You're welcome. See the two of you in two days.

This is an example of a physician working with a relatively "easy" patient. Is this physician practicing psychiatry? "Behavioral medicine" perhaps would be a more descriptive term. The patient is a genital character. She does not present with features suggesting an axis II diagnosis. Even so, the physician's interviewing skill facilitates the therapeutic sequence. As skill increases, so does success with "difficult" patients. Compliance increases. Patient satisfaction is enhanced, and patient outcome measures improve.

# THE THERAPEUTIC SEQUENCE AND DIFFICULT PATIENTS

With relatively healthy people, genital characters or near-genital characters, the process of the therapeutic sequence tends to move quite smoothly, especially for experienced clinicians who have incorporated the model into the way they typically function with patients consistent with their specialty. An example was provided in the previous section. You may find it useful to review that example again before proceeding (refer also to Fig. 2-1).

Problems tend to develop in the areas of establishing congruence, establishing consensus, and obtaining concurrence relative to the contract. This is particularly the case when working with patients who have axis II diagnoses or have major features of one or more personality disorders. Proceeding toward a positive therapeutic outcome then is simply more difficult, whether the patient is seeing a surgeon, an internist, a family physician, or a psychiatrist.

## Congruence Problems

### Condition 1

The patient presents with little or no objective or subjective evidence of a distressing, dis-easing emotion, but the absence is not appropriate to the situation. The patient talks in a fashion that seems to avoid the expression of feeling, even when asked directly. Often, the patient uses language that seems to serve the purpose of distancing himself or herself from what a genital character would acknowledge as a distressing event. The terms "denial" or "repression," among others, are used to understand such psychopathology. (Advances in neurobiology have demonstrated brain mechanisms that can be correlated with these behaviors, at least in part.)

When such patients approach an affective interface, they often shift talking about themselves in the first person to second person, or even third person. Instead of saying, "I think . . . ," they say, "You would think

. . . ," "A person would think . . . ," "A good Christian believes . . . ." By affective interface, we mean the boundary between a topic that might be assumed to be somewhat neutral in feeling tone and one in which significant accompanying affect or emotion would be expected.

**EXAMPLES**

Assume you are the physician to a 32-year-old woman who has given birth to a stillborn boy. You know that she and her husband planned for the pregnancy, wanted the baby, and both have prepared for the baby's arrival. You have noticed that she seems to present very little, if any, objective evidence for distress, whether sadness or anger, even when asked about her baby.

Assume you are the physician to a 37-year-old man. He has a family history of rectal cancer with deaths in several family members. He makes an appointment, stating that he simply needs "a regular checkup." In talking with you, however, he informs you that in the past week he has noted bloody stools. Nonetheless, he presents no objective evidence for fear, nor do his verbal statements suggest subjective awareness of anxiety.

In the first example, one would expect a grief response; in the second, a normal fear response. These two patients, when asked directly how they feel about the event, tend to reply by talking about what they think or what they believe. Similar examples could be provided for an expected normal disgust reaction or an expected normal anger reaction.

*Interventions* here include such statements as, "I understand that's what you think, but I'm interested in knowing how you *feel*." "When you think that, how do you feel?" "When you imagine that, how do you feel?" "I'm making a distinction between thinking and feeling. Could you tell me how you feel?" "What do you think most people would feel in this situation?" The skilled physician or skilled therapist, by asking these questions, is moving toward the key intervention, something like, "*How do you stop yourself from feeling?*"

The reader at this point might review axis II personality diagnoses, perhaps bringing to mind particular patients that fit this condition.

## Condition 2

The patient presents with considerable subjective evidence. They use words indicating an awareness of feeling within themselves. However, they present little objective evidence, that is, these patients do not look the way they say they feel. The price of such a tendency is that the listener, including their physician, tends to discount the verbal expression of feeling. Studies have demonstrated repeatedly that patients who complain of pain but do not appear to be in pain tend to be ignored. The term, "inhibition," describes this psychopathology. Some patients, somatizers, talk about the physiologic accompaniments to anxiety, anger, or sadness but without speaking about the emotions, *per se*. They often describe these symptoms in considerable detail, appointment after appointment.

They may build a very thick chart over months and years! Others, psychologizers, may talk at some length directly about feeling, about emotions, appointment after appointment. Condition 2 is more common in primary care than condition 1. Both are difficult.

**EXAMPLE**

Assume you are the primary care physician to a 46-year-old woman who is returning to you for follow-up after a hysterectomy for uterine fibroids 2 months ago. She states, "I'm furious with the surgeon. He promised me I'd be free of pain when I recovered. And to be honest I'm kind of aggravated with you." All this is said in a flat tone of voice and without objective evidence for anger that matches the intensity of feeling suggested in the semantics of her sentence.

*Interventions* here are to ask the patient, "Do you feel this way, now?" "When you feel this way, what does it usually mean?" "If you didn't tell me you were feeling this way, how would I know?" "When do you suppose, you felt this way before?" These questions move toward the key intervention, "*How do you stop yourself from showing (such-and-such a feeling)?*" and beyond that, "What consequences do you suppose there are for you to feel this way, even though you do not look this way?"

Again, the reader may wish to review axis II diagnoses and bring to mind particular experiences with patients.

## Condition 3

The patient presents objective evidence of a distressing emotion but little subjective evidence for awareness. This is the most common condition of the three presented by patients in primary care settings. "Denial," again, is a term commonly used to describe this variety of psychopathology. These patients talk with very much the same semantic structure in their sentences as those in the first condition. In contrast, however, there are facial expressions or hand or foot gestures presenting objective evidence.

**EXAMPLE**

Assume you are the physician to a 29-year-old man who is seeing you for severe tension headaches. When asked how these affect his life, he responds, "They are getting in the way of my doing my work. I'm a loan officer and damn near every day just when I need to present my justifications to the Vice President I seem to get one. And I need my wits about me because he's basically impossible to deal with." Objective facial evidence of anger is clearly present. Subjective evidence is missing in his statement.

*Interventions* might include, "How do you feel about the Vice President?" "Are you aware of how you look when you talk about him?" "Have others ever commented that you look irritated or annoyed when you talk about (this subject)?" "If you saw someone who looked like this [describe or demonstrate], what would you assume they were feeling?" Here, after appropriate preliminary work, the key intervention is something like, "*How do you stop yourself from knowing how you feel?*"

Once more, ask yourself what kind of patients present this picture.

# Establishing Consensus

Once congruence is established or incongruence is noted and acknowledged by the patient, at least to some degree, then the following guidelines may be helpful in **identifying** the **precipitating stress**.

1. Begin by assuming the **usual linkage**; for fear, look for a stress in the past or in the present suggesting the threat of injury; for anger, the stress of frustration; for sadness, the possibility of loss. Specifically, ask the patient, "How do you understand this feeling?" or "How do you account for this feeling?" In their response, assume that patients are on the right track.
2. The right track may be signaled by the **appearance of a new primary emotion**. The right track may be only partially hidden by use of verbal body language. The right track may be buried within the subtleties of the semantics of the sentence. The right track may be suggested by a train of associations.
3. Many times, patients respond that they are not certain or that they do not know. Inviting patients to "guess" is sometimes a useful instruction. Their **guess is often an indicator** that they are on the right track.
4. Consensus is facilitated by helping the patient talk in complete sentences. We will discuss this later, in particular, in the paragraphs dealing with in the transformations of deletion, generalization, and distortion (see page 109).
5. **Helping the patient make connections** is the key. Until the patient makes connections, both the patient and the physician are uncertain about the precipitating stress. Toward that end, note the **all-purpose sentence** in Figure 2-2.

# Contracting and Concurrence

Begin contracting by **eliciting the chief expectation**, as previously discussed. The patient's expectation and yours may be similar. Concurrence is readily accomplished.

The expectations of some patients, however, turn out to be almost magical in quality: "All I want you to do is make me happy." "I want you to give me something so I don't feel so nervous." "I want you to do something so I'll never hurt again."

Another group of patients present expectations that, although not magical, are at considerable variance with what is necessary to do to determine the underlying problem or what is necessary to implement an effective intervention. The cue of how to proceed with a specific individual relates specifically to understanding the dynamics inherent in your diagnosis of them as a person.

With this process, the strategy for intervention often becomes almost self-evident, not only to the physician but to the patient. Invite the patient to participate in the decision making. This may begin with a question such as, "Well, given our understanding of the problem, what ideas do you have of how *you* might proceed, and

**Making Connections**

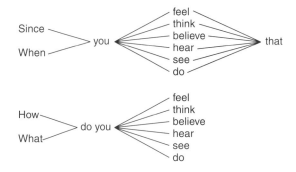

Examples:
  "When your husband does that, how do you feel?"
  "When you feel like you're getting a headache,
      what do you think?"
  "When she says that, how does she look?"

**Figure 2-2.**
The all-purpose sentence.

what ideas do you have as to how *we* might proceed?" Once again, recall the characteristics of effective physicians—they are skilled in involving the patient in problem solving.

# NOSOLOGY AND STAGES OF COGNITION

Having brought certain critical **concepts** to the patient encounter, having performed the **attitudinal** task in which the physician has come to know his or her emotional response tendencies, psychological needs, belief system biases, and **perceptual** priorities, having accurately seen and heard the patient, having noticed or elicited pertinent information, and having interacted skillfully **interpersonally** and with an appropriate communication style, the physician then proceeds with the **nosologic** task. The physician proceeds to make a disease diagnosis as well as a patient diagnosis.

The preceding is all very logical and sequential. Perhaps, it is even appropriate for pedagogy to be organized in this fashion. But of course, the brain does not work this way. The physician's brain is already organized to recognize patterns long before medical school, residency, and medical practice.

During the process of becoming an effective physician, there are certain sequential stages of cognition. The first is the **stage of propositional thinking**, and is characteristic of first- and second-year medical students (Table 2-8). They work laboriously to acquire an understanding of basic body processes—this feature is linked to this feature, this biochemical response triggers the next, and so forth. When asked, for example, how they might account for an elevated body temperature in a particular patient, they typically go through an elaborate sequential description. However, already by the second year, this elaborate propositional thinking is considerably truncated. They tend to respond to the same question by stating, "The patient has a bacterial infection and in the presence of a bacterial infection you expect a fever." The network has been **abridged**. Note that the experienced physician thinks the other way around—"When I am in the presence of a patient with fever, I consider a bacterial infection."

Beginning in the third year and certainly throughout the early years of residency training, the principal cognitive work is elabo-

---

**TABLE 2-8.**

**Sequential Stages of Cognition**

| Stage Theory Clinical Reasoning | Curriculum | Cognitive Work | USMLE Evaluation |
|---|---|---|---|
| Propositional networks | Medical student | | |
| | I  Biology | Body process elucidation | |
| | II  Pathophysiology | | Step 1 |
| Abridged networks | | | |
| | III  Organ system nosology | Symptom explanation | |
| | IV  Generic nosology | | Step 2 |
| Illness scripts | Postgraduate years | | |
| | I  Illnesses | Script search, selection and verification | |
| | II | | Step 3 |
| Instance scripts | | | |
| | III | Management selection | |
| | IV  Specific kinds of people who have specific kinds of illnesses | | |
| | V | | |
| | VI | | |

rating on what are known as **illness scripts**. "Here then, is a particular set of symptoms and findings to which can be attached a diagnostic label." Most of what has been learned and retained so far has been accomplished by what is known as **semantic memory**. This knowledge comes, in considerable measure, by simply memorizing a typical textbook of medicine. It is augmented, of course, by seeing patients. Increasingly, what is being used is pattern recognition. "This sounds and looks like gallbladder disease." Many physicians stay stuck, so to speak, at this level. With experience, **episodic memory** is brought into play. The competent physician literally has in his or her memory an instance of a particular patient with a particular personality with a particular illness that responded to medical intervention in a particular way. "And now I see in front of me another patient of similar category." This pattern transcends an illness script. It is an **instance script**. Feeling is typically attached to or included with episodic memory; the experienced physician is now responding to this kind of gestalt.

Hence, effective physicians in their patient encounters have a very early diagnostic impression. The impression is made consciously, but effective physicians do not deify their diagnosis. They pay particular attention to their surprise when they see or hear a piece of evidence that does not fit. They rule diseases in, not other diseases out. This approach is usually more accurate and clearly more cost effective. These physicians say to themselves and make a report to others something like this, "The patient *said*, 'I have this pain in my chest which goes down my arm when I walk up the stairs.'" These physicians do not say, "The patient *claims* to have chest pain that radiates down the left arm," or "This patient *admits* that the chest pain radiates down her left arm." The verbs "claim" and "admit" suggest the following, internal, attitudinal set. "This patient is saying something that doesn't fit my gestalt, therefore this patient is only claiming something that I really don't believe is there." Or, conversely, "I managed to get data from this patient that fits my gestalt; I got this patient to admit this symptom." Both views suggest a deification of diagnosis. Errors in disease diagnosis and errors in patient diagnosis lead to failures in patient management. Chapters 3 through 12 discuss our current nosology. The outline follows *DSM-IV*.

# Chapter 3

# Disorders Usually Presenting in Infancy, Childhood, or Adolescence

Mental retardation is defined as lower than average general intelligence with resulting deficits or impairments in adaptive behavior. The four subtypes—**mild**, **moderate**, **severe**, and **profound**—have prognostic implications. Milder cases often are not diagnosed until scholastic difficulty is noted in grade school. People with this level of disability may attain a sixth-grade performance level. The moderate group is also educable, perhaps to the fourth-grade level. The severe are trainable to some degree; the profound require custodial care.

From 1% to 3% of the population of the United States is mentally retarded. The term **primary** designates those instances in which no specific etiology can be identified or reasonably postulated. This constitutes the largest group, approximately 30% of the patient population. They usually have no other symptoms; there may be family history. All others are referred to as **secondary**. Perinatal infections, especially viral, and early childhood encephalitides cause about 20% of cases. Prematurity and birth trauma may account for another 20%. Causes may be categorized under **prenatal** factors, for example, phenylketonuria, Gaucher's disease, cretinism, Hurler's syndrome (gargoylism), and Down's syndrome (mongolism). About 10% of persons who are mentally retarded suffer from mongolism. **Perinatal** factors are a second category (e.g., prematurity, birth injury, or kernicterus). Examples of **postnatal** factors include viral meningoencephalitis, lead poisoning, and malnutrition. Sociocultural factors may play a role. Emotional problems and environmental deprivation may result in a picture sometimes called pseudomental retardation, a particularly important diagnosis to make.

Prevention of retardation should be a special concern of all health professionals. Treatment should focus on etiologic factors whenever possible. In the main, treatment means bringing appropriate support to the family and to the child, with particular attention to special classes in school or appropriate institutional or custodial care to those instances of profound retardation.

## LEARNING AND COMMUNICATION DISORDERS

Formerly termed "academic skills disorders," the subclassification of learning disorders includes reading disorder, mathematics disorder, and disorder of written expression. Communication disorders refer to **spoken language**. With language, the problem may be primarily expressive or receptive or relating to articulation. The older term "dyslexia" no longer appears as a diagnosis in *DSM-IV*.

These disorders tend to occur in children who have average or higher than average intellectual endowment and achievement in non-language-related subjects. There are few if any positive signs on classic neurologic examination, and these are of the so-called "soft" variety. The diagnosis may be suspected by teachers. It should also be considered by physicians in children who may present with a variety of psychophysiologic, behavioral, and emotional symptoms that develop secondary to the stress of attempting to cope with what has heretofore been an unrecognized problem by peers, parents, and teachers. Learning disorders are quite **common**. What happens to these children depends on the support they get from their family, the kind of remedial help they receive from their school, and their own capacity to learn coping techniques to compensate for the specific deficit. These disorders are to be distinguished from inadequate schooling, impaired vision or hearing, mental retardation, or infantile autism.

## ATTENTION DEFICIT–HYPERACTIVITY DISORDER

Attention deficit–hyperactivity disorder is characterized by **inattention**, for example, having difficulty concentrating on school work; **impulsivity**; and, sometimes, **hyperactivity**. Onset is before age **7** years. The diagnosis should not be made unless symptoms have been present for at least 6 months. Parents report excessive activity and short attention span. Similar reports come from teachers. Current thinking about etiology points to central nervous system maturational factors interacting with environmental stresses. Treatment is directed toward parental counseling, education, environmental manipulation, and usually medication with methylphenidate or pemoline. Aspects of this disorder may persist into adulthood.

## CONDUCT DISORDERS

The diagnosis of conduct disorder may be made in patients younger than 18 years of age when there is a repetitive and persistent pattern of conduct for at least 6 months in which the basic rights of others are either ignored or violated. The behaviors may be **aggressive**, for example, physical violence against property or persons, or theft; or **nonaggressive**, for example, a recurring and chronic tendency to violate rules, or lie. Another important distinction is whether the disorder is of the **undersocialized** or **socialized** variety. The undersocialized group fails to establish normal bonds of affection with others. In the socialized variety, there is evidence of emotional bonding or attachment to others, frequently to peers, often with considerable loyalty to the peer group (this variety previously was called "group delinquent reaction"). This disorder commonly is found in the slums of our large cities where security and self-esteem are centered in antisocial acts supported by peers. Etiology relates primarily to faulty parental attitudes, poor child-rearing practices, emotional conflicts, and a variety of sociocultural factors. Intervention follows accordingly.

Somewhat related is what is now termed an **oppositional deficit disorder**.

# ANXIETY DISORDERS

The **separation anxiety disorder** is characterized by manifestations of excessive anxiety clearly relating to separation from a significant person to whom the child feels attached. Symptoms should be present for at least 2 weeks before this diagnosis is made.

There are a variety of other attachment disorders of infancy and childhood, all less common.

It should be remembered that **phobias** often have their onset in childhood and adolescence, as does the **generalized anxiety disorder**.

If anxiety symptoms are present for a relatively short period of time and relate to a specific stress, the diagnosis of an **adjustment reaction** is usually more appropriate. Here, the symptoms persist beyond the stress and are to be distinguished from what might be termed as a normal fear response. In older children, this tends to be symptomatic of an underlying neurotic disorder, especially when responses are not **age appropriate**. Various psychological and counseling techniques are indicated. Antianxiety medication usually should be avoided except in special cases and for brief periods of time.

# EATING DISORDERS

**Pica** refers to the eating of nonnutritive substances repeatedly for at least 1 month.

**Bulimia nervosa** refers to recurrent episodes of binge eating of large quantities of food, often with termination by self-induced vomiting, repeated attempts to lose weight by severely restrictive diets or purging through laxatives, marked weight fluctuation, awareness that the eating pattern is abnormal, and a fear of being unable to stop, coupled with an overconcern about body shape and weight together with depression and self-deprecatory thoughts. This group is to be distinguished from those with anorexia nervosa. Both may develop during early adulthood.

**Anorexia nervosa**, more common in adolescent girls than boys, presents with all of the physiologic findings of what is essentially self-induced starvation. The syndrome is not related to a known physical illness. The diagnosis should be considered when there is weight loss of at least 15% of the original body weight, a refusal to maintain body weight over a minimum normal for the age and height, and when there is an intense fear of becoming obese, or a disturbance of body image. These patients may report feeling fat when objectively they are almost emaciated. Many feel quite energetic and may even engage in body-building exercises. Amenorrhea is common. Without effective intervention, there is significant mortality to this syndrome. Hospitalization may be necessary as a life-saving procedure.

Intervention is often complicated because there is a tendency on the part of the patient and the family to deny the presence of serious psychological difficulties. With therapy, severe conflicts regarding dependency and sexuality usually become apparent. No medication, to date, has been shown to be consistently effective.

# STEREOTYPED MOVEMENT DISORDERS

**Tics** are to be distinguished from choreiform, dystonic, and athetoid movements. They are characterized as recurrent, involuntary, repetitive, purposeless movements. The patient is able to suppress the movement voluntarily for minutes to hours. A tic disorder may be subclassified either as **transient**, that is, lasting at least a month but no more than a year, or **chronic**. The syndrome is usually thought to be psychogenic in origin, and hence counseling and psychotherapy are indicated.

A separate syndrome, relatively rare, is **Tourette's disorder**. The tics involve multiple muscle groups. There are frequently vocal tics as well, sometimes with compulsive and stereotyped coprolalia. Here also, the movements may be suppressed for minutes to hours and symptoms vary in intensity over weeks to months. The criteria for diagnosis include the presence of symptoms for more than a year. Organic disease of the central nervous system has consistently been suspected as playing a role in this disorder. To date, there is no reliable effective treatment, although haloperidol has been reported to be helpful in some cases.

The **stereotypic movement disorder** is characterized by repetitive, seemingly driven, nonfunctional behavior (e.g., body rocking or head bending).

## OTHER DISORDERS WITH PHYSICAL MANIFESTATIONS

**Stuttering** is a syndrome over which there is considerable controversy regarding etiology and treatment. However, in some cases, psychological factors clearly play a role and psychological intervention is effective. In others, such is not the case.

**Functional enuresis** and **functional encopresis** are not caused by a physical disorder, by definition. They are manifested by the repeated, involuntary voiding of urine by day or night or the voluntary or involuntary passage of feces. One or both may be present. There should be a history of at least one event per month in children older than age 4 or 5 years for this diagnosis. Eighty to 90% of children are dry, that is, not enuretic by age 4.5 years. By age 18 years, the percentage of enuretics in the general population drops to about 2%. With enuresis, there is a growing opinion that causation in many cases may relate more to maturational or developmental factors than to classic psychodynamic considerations. Encopresis is much less common. When these symptoms appear transiently in essentially healthy young children in response to a specific stressful life event, the diagnosis of an **adjustment reaction** is more appropriate.

**Sleepwalking** and **sleep terrors** occur during non-REM (rapid eye movement) periods of sleep, in contrast to nightmares. Nightmares have psychological significance, but sleep terrors relate more to maturational lags in central nervous system development than to psychodynamic factors, and reassurance and counseling to parents are in order.

## PERVASIVE DEVELOPMENTAL DISORDERS

The child with **infantile autism** seems to dwell within his or her own world, out of reach. He or she lacks responsiveness to other people. There is a gross deficit in language development. Responses to environment are bizarre. Onset is before age 3 years. There is considerable controversy about etiology, but a recent emphasis is on biologic factors. Normal siblings are common. Patterns of interaction seen between parents and such children probably relate more to the parents' reaction to the frustration of dealing with such a child, and should ordinarily be viewed in that context rather than seeing the interaction as pathogenic for the syndrome. There are other, less common pervasive developmental disorders as well. (It should be noted that schizophrenia can have its onset in childhood.) These diagnostic categories are relatively uncommon.

# OTHER ISSUES ASSOCIATED WITH INFANCY, CHILDHOOD, AND ADOLESCENCE

Most children and adolescents who present to health professionals with psychological problems do *not* fall into one of the previously mentioned categories. First, there are **age-appropriate behaviors** that are of concern to parents, for whom educational techniques and reassurance are indicated. Examples include the expected stranger anxiety of 8 months, the oppositional behaviors of the 18- to 36-month-old toddler, the transient phobias of the 4- or 5-year-old, and the insecurity and identity issues of early adolescence.

Second, many responses in children are most appropriately diagnosed as **adjustment disorders** in response to such environmental stresses as illness, hospitalization, surgery, divorce of parents, birth of siblings, loss of a playmate, difficulty in school, and so forth. These symptoms tend to be transient, especially when the child is given support in a system by concerned others. The symptoms may be regressive to earlier behaviors, such as thumb-sucking or wetting the bed. Or, depending on the age, the symptoms may be manifested as a conduct disturbance of one kind or another, or as that group of symptoms that have been called neurotic traits.

Persistent neurotic behaviors with evidence for psychopathology in children or adolescents should be diagnosed as one of the disorders to be outlined and described later in this text. Schizophrenia essentially indistinguishable in onset from that seen in young adulthood can also develop in late childhood and early adolescence. Finally, many symptoms presented by children fall into the psychophysiologic disorder category, and are now categorized under "psychological factors affecting physical condition."

Other issues of considerable concern to primary care physicians, child psychiatrists, and other health professionals are such psychological problems as maternal deprivation, child abuse, the cultural aspects of delinquent behavior, and substance abuse in children and adolescents.

# Chapter 4

# Disorders Associated with Cognitive Impairments

A group of brain syndromes, caused in general by specific general medical conditions or related to specific substances, is fairly well defined and recognizable. Each has multiple possible etiologies. These syndromes are described first; more specific disorders linked to more specific etiologies are discussed later.

## DELIRIUM

Delirium develops over a relatively short period of time, usually hours or days, and tends to fluctuate over the course of the day. Symptoms include clouding of consciousness, disorientation, reduced ability to focus or sustain attention, memory impairment, frequent perceptual disturbances such as illusions or hallucinations, speech that may be incoherent, a disturbed sleep–wakefulness cycle, and either increased or decreased psychomotor activity. With this syndrome, as with all those that follow, there is reason to believe, based on history, physical examination, or laboratory tests, that a **specific organic factor** may be etiologically related to the disturbance.

Delirium is to be differentiated from acute schizophrenic illness. In general, acute visual hallucinations should suggest a delirium. Auditory hallucinations are more characteristic of schizophrenia. The type of thinking disorder typical of schizophrenia tends to be absent with organic delirium. **Clouding of consciousness**, typical of delirium, is absent in schizophrenia.

## DEMENTIA

With dementia, in contrast to delirium, there is not a clouding of consciousness, and **symptoms usually develop over a long period of time**. There is evidence for loss of intellectual ability, memory difficulties (especially for recent memory), impairment of abstract thinking with substitution of concrete thinking, and impairment of judgment. Emotional lability is common. Other disturbances of higher cortical function such as aphasia, apraxia, and agnosia may be present. Often a personality change that tends to be an accentuation of premorbid personality traits is noted. Especially in elderly people, severe depression may be confused with dementia, and vice versa. It is critical that this differential diagnosis be made because depression, with treatment, tends to have a better prognosis.

## AMNESTIC SYNDROME
With the amnestic syndrome, there is both short-term memory impairment and long-term memory impairment, but in the absence of clouding of consciousness, as in delirium, and in the absence of general loss of major intellectual functions, as in dementia. There is also impairment in the ability to learn new information.

## INTOXICATION
This term is used when a substance-specific syndrome develops after the recent ingestion of that substance. Maladaptive behaviors such as disorientation, impaired judgment, and belligerence result from the impact of the substance on the central nervous system (CNS). Intoxication has many features comparable to delirium.

## WITHDRAWAL
This refers to the development of a substance-specific syndrome after the cessation or reduction of intake of that substance, especially when it was previously used by the person to induce a state of intoxication. Clinical features are similar to delirium or to other of the various organic syndromes.

## DELUSIONAL SYNDROME
In the absence of clouding of consciousness, loss of intellectual abilities, and prominent hallucinations, delusions are the prominent clinical feature.

## HALLUCINOSIS
Persistent or recurring hallucinations are the predominant feature.

## MOOD SYNDROME
Most prominent here is a mood disturbance, either of the manic or depressive variety.

## ANXIETY SYNDROME
This syndrome is characterized by either panic attacks or generalized anxiety. There is evidence of a specific organic factor etiologically.

## PERSONALITY SYNDROME
This syndrome is characterized by a marked change in behavior or personality. Here, as with the organic hallucinosis and affective

syndromes, there is absence of clouding of consciousness, as in delirium, and absence of significant loss of intellectual abilities, as in dementia.

**DEPENDENCE**

Dependence on a specific substance is characterized by tolerance—an increasing amount of substance necessary to maintain the intoxication or the desired effect; withdrawal—discontinuation or decreased ingestion of the substance is associated with a characteristic pattern of physiologic or behavioral effects; and often undesired or unsuccessful efforts to discontinue or control use, increasing effort, time, and money invested in the activity to the detriment of other activities, and persistence of use in spite of deleterious physical or psychological effects.

**ABUSE**

Abuse is the term used when there is an absence of tolerance and withdrawal. Otherwise, the characteristics are similar to dependence.

# DISORDERS

## Alzheimer's Disease (Senile Dementia, Presenile Dementia)

Although this disease may begin at any age, it usually develops insidiously later in life. The final features are usually those of dementia, but the disorder may begin as an amnestic syndrome. The dementia may be accompanied by delirium, delusions, or depression. From 5% to 15% of people older than 65 years of age have dementia of this category. Throughout the world, this disorder results in one of our most significant medical and sociologic problems. The precise etiology is unknown. In some families there is a hereditary factor. The transmitter acetylcholine has been implicated in some studies. Neuronal degeneration occurs, producing amyloid deposits and neurofibrillary tangles. Early in the illness, the patient may be aware of losing previous capacity and may react to this loss with grief or depression. However, later in the course of the illness, patients often show little indication of being aware of their problem.

## Multi-infarct Dementia

Most of the statements made about Alzheimer's disease (above) apply to this category of dementia as well. The syndrome is secondary to multiple infarcts. Symptoms may appear over a shorter period of time and not so insidiously as with Alzheimer's disease. Diagnosis is made by history and course, and later by pathologic findings. Imaging studies are useful for diagnosis. Arteriosclerotic dementia is a diagnosis that is being used less and less as evidence increases that these so-called cases, when closely examined, tend to be either Alzheimer's disease or multi-infarct dementia.

## Disorders Induced by Alcohol

Alcohol can produce the whole spectrum of what have been called organic brain syndromes in the past and are described in the first section of this chapter. In addition to the very common **alcohol intoxication**, there is also **alcohol idiosyncratic intoxication**, in which there is a marked behavioral change to behavior atypical of the person when not drinking, secondary to an ingestion of an amount of alcohol insufficient to induce intoxication in most people.

The **alcohol withdrawal syndrome** (delirium tremens) is well known and may or may not be accompanied by delirium. The syndrome develops within 1 week of withdrawal and is characterized by a coarse tremor of the hands or tongue, frequently nausea and vomiting, weakness, anxiety, depressed mood or irritability, orthostatic hypotension, and various signs of autonomic hyperactivity. Although withdrawal may be limited to these symptoms, a delirium may be superimposed, as may seizures. This illness without vigorous medical treatment has significant mortality.

**Alcohol hallucinosis** may be confused with an acute schizophrenic illness. On withdrawal from alcohol, usually within 48 hours, there are vivid hallucinations, predominantly auditory. In contrast to delirium tremens, there is no clouding of consciousness.

The **alcohol amnestic disorder** (blackouts) is a pathognomonic indicator of alcohol dependency. Prolonged, heavy ingestion of alcohol may also result in *dementia. Abuse* and *dependence* are discussed later.

## Disorders Induced by Other Central Nervous System-Active Agents

**Barbiturates** may result in intoxication and withdrawal syndromes with or without delirium. The same can be said of almost any similarly acting sedative, including the **benzodiazepines**.

**Opioid intoxication** is usually accompanied by pupillary constriction and a change in mood, that is, euphoria, dysphoria, or apathy. **Opioid withdrawal** is characterized by pupillary dilation, lacrimation, rhinorrhea, piloerection, sweating, diarrhea, yawning, mild hypertension, tachycardia, insomnia, and fever.

**Cocaine intoxication**, in addition to physical symptoms and signs of autonomic nervous system hyperactivity, often includes symptoms of psychomotor agitation or elation with elements of grandiosity or hypervigilance.

**Amphetamines** or similarly acting sympathomimetic agents can result in intoxication, delirium, and withdrawal. The intoxication is similar to that of cocaine. The delirium and especially the accompanying delusional disorder may be similar to an acute schizophrenic illness, with rapidly developing persecutory delusions as a prominent feature. Withdrawal is characterized by depressed mood, disturbed sleep, and increased dreaming. **Phencyclidine** or similarly acting agents may result in intoxication or delirium. The **hallucinogens** may produce a hallucinosis, a delusional disorder, or an affective disorder. Perceptual changes are characteristic of the hallucinosis, with synesthesias, hallucinations, illusions, depersonalization, or merely the report of subjective intensification of perceptions, all occurring in a state of full wakefulness and alertness. Again, physiologic symptoms and signs, mainly of hyperactivity within the autonomic nervous system, frequently accompany this disorder.

**Cannabis intoxication** is characterized by tachycardia, euphoria or apathy, a sensation of slowed time, and a subjective intensification of perceptions. Physical symptoms and signs often include increased appetite, dry mouth, and conjunctival injection. Cannabis can also result in a delusional disorder, but this does not persist beyond 6 hours after cessation of its use. Many other substances can produce intoxication and withdrawal, including **caffeine** and **tobacco** in sufficient doses. A major addicting drug in tobacco is **nicotine**, and the major withdrawal symptom is an intense craving for the resumption of smoking.

## Disorders Secondary to Other Etiologies

### Disturbances Associated with the Circulatory System

In addition to multi-infarct dementia and arteriosclerotic dementia, circulatory system disturbances can result in a variety of organic brain syndromes. Acute cerebral infarction may include a delirium-like syndrome in addition to focal signs. Bilateral lesions of the hippocampus may result in an amnestic syndrome. Any hypoxic state, whatever the etiology, can accentuate delirium or superimpose on dementia an increased confusion-like state. Of particular interest are the confusional states manifested after cardiac surgery.

### Metabolic and Endocrine Disorders

In the category of **metabolic and endocrine disorders**, *delirium* is a feature of hepatic, uremic, and hypoglycemic encephalopathies, as is diabetic ketoacidosis. Symptoms of anxiety and emotional instability, even delirium, may accompany acute intermittent porphyria. Endocrine disorders, whether involving the thyroid, the parathyroid, or the adrenal gland, can be accompanied by changes in personality and impairment of mental functions and memory. Myxedema may mimic depression or early dementia.

**Huntington's chorea**, although relatively rare, is a hereditary disorder characterized by choreiform movements and dementia that begins in adult life.

**Normal-pressure hydrocephalus** may be characterized by a progressive dementia. These patients have enlarged ventricles but normal cerebrospinal fluid pressure. There may be associated gait disturbances.

**Brain trauma** can present acutely as a delirium and over time as a Korsakoff-like syndrome showing elements of amnesia and confabulation. Delayed sequelae, depending on the nature of the trauma, and whether the trauma is repetitive, can result in the whole spectrum of brain syndromes.

**Infections of the CNS or systemic infections** frequently include features of delirium. If the CNS infection is more chronic, a dementia can result, the classic example being the general paralysis of the insane secondary to syphilis (dementia paralytica). Neuropsychiatric complications in patients with acquired immunodeficiency syndrome are common and of increasing concern.

**Organic brain disorders** may be associated with intracranial neoplasia.

Certain of these disorders may be associated with **epilepsy**. After a grand mal seizure, the patient's confused state has features of delirium. Temporal lobe seizures may be difficult to differentiate from dissociative reactions. Between seizures, some patients with epilepsy may show brief, interseizure psychotic episodes; most of these occur in cases of psychomotor epilepsy.

# TREATMENT

## Organic Brain Syndromes

Treatment of the organic brain syndromes should **focus on the underlying etiology**. The more specific medical treatments are not reviewed here, but certain guidelines regarding general management are made.

With delirium in particular, general medical support measures are indicated—fluids, electrolyte balance, nutrition. Sedatives and all other nonvital drugs should be discontinued. Precautions against suicide should be considered. Human contacts, especially friends, should be encouraged. Friends and personnel can be extremely helpful in providing reassuring and orienting verbal input. When the patient is awake, the light should be on in the room. Avoid mechanical restraints if at all possible. Urge the patient to accept their hallucinations as bad dreams. If medication becomes necessary to manage agitated or aggressive, destructive behavior, avoid barbiturates, and consider haloperidol or chlorpromazine. Chlordiazepoxide is often helpful with alcohol withdrawal syndromes.

With the **dementias**, in addition to instituting a specific treatment aimed at a known etiology, general treatment should focus on consulting with the patient's family, providing a protected physical and social environment, maintaining activity, and avoiding social or physical isolation or immobilization. **Appropriate supportive psychotherapeutic** and **environmental maneuvers** can sometimes result in dramatic improvement. Again, **depression** can be superimposed on a dementia or be confused with it. Any medical illness can intensify the symptoms of dementia. Some patients with "dementia" improve dramatically when unnecessary medications are withdrawn or inappropriately high doses of medication are reduced.

## Substance Abuse and Dependence

Clinically, indicators of alcoholism (alcohol dependence) include a steady increase in alcohol intake or drinking sprees, solitary drinking, early morning drinking, and occurrence of blackouts. Operationally, a person may be considered alcoholic if unable to stop the consumption of alcohol despite the fact that drinking is clearly causing physical illness or repeated difficulty with employers, family, or the police.

Two types of alcoholism have been characterized: **type I**, with passive dependent or anxious personality traits, has its onset usually after age 25 years; **type II**, with antisocial traits, has its onset before age 25 years. Multiple therapeutic approaches are used, including alcohol treatment programs in hospital and community settings, psychotherapeutic intervention in selected patients, the use of conditioned reflex treatment involving disulfiram (Antabuse), and Alcoholics Anonymous and other group therapies or support systems. Initially, denial is a major mechanism seen in most alcoholics. Many are experts in self-destruction and are skilled in manipulating their environment to provide a continuing source of alcohol. Many physicians have severe countertransference problems with these patients. Nonetheless, if the illness is viewed as a chronic one and intervention is persistent, the prognosis for many can be quite good.

The abuse of and dependence on different drugs vary from time to time and from country to country. Many addicts state they take drugs to experience euphoria, to feel "normal," or to overcome states of depression. Narcotic addicts have a wide range of personality characteristics, but many are described as immature, impulsive, and emotionally unstable. Treatment programs, as with alcohol treatment programs, are multifaceted. Addicts Anonymous is modeled after Alcoholics Anonymous. Substitute programs, in which, for example, methadone is substituted for heroin, are widely used but still seen by many as experimental and subject to increasing criticism in recent years. In the clinical setting, nalorphine, an antagonist, may be used to test for evidence of readdiction. A current trend for people who abuse drugs is involvement with more than one agent.

Successful treatment of **tobacco addiction** is of considerable import given the disabilities imposed by smoking over time and the mortality from these disorders (see Table 2-1). Treatment programs designed with the same principles as those outlined previously have been shown to be helpful. Studies show that "quit rates" tend to improve when there is strong motivation on the part of the smoker to discontinue the habit, when the patient's physician strongly recommends such cessation and continues support for cessation even with lapses, when the smoker is surrounded by a system in support of such cessation, and at least in some instances when the program includes appropriate use of the nicotine patch technique. The active patch improves quit rates even without behavioral counseling, but intensive counseling appears to double such quit rates. These rates, however, are not improved significantly with the use of the patch beyond 8 or 10 weeks, at least as shown by some studies.

Chapter 5

# Schizophrenia and Other Psychotic Disorders

## Schizophrenia

Schizophrenia is one of the psychoses. A salient feature is a defect in reality testing that may be manifest in the schizophrenic's relationship to self, to the objects in the world, or to others. Bleuler distinguished between primary and secondary symptoms. The primary or fundamental symptoms include disturbances in associations (e.g., loosening, blocking, neologisms), disturbances in affect (disharmony or incongruity between ideas and emotion), ambivalence (multiple and contradictory feelings of extreme degree), and autism (preoccupation with self). Secondary or accessory symptoms include hallucinations, delusions, and bizarre behavior.

Modern criteria emphasize the **thought disorder**. Occasionally, the disorder may be so profound that speech is incoherent. Examination more commonly reveals tangentiality, loosening of association, or poverty of speech content. A mixture of autistic and concrete thinking is common. This may be accompanied by blunted or inappropriate affect. Disorganized behavior is common. Delusions are bizarre in content; they may be somatic, grandiose, religious, nihilistic, or persecutory. Hallucinations, especially auditory hallucinations, may be evident. When one or more sets of these symptoms is accompanied by deterioration of previous level of functioning, whether relating to taking care of self, to significant others, or to educational activities or work, and when these signs have been present for at least 6 months, the diagnosis is warranted.

Differential diagnoses include the organic mental disorders and manic–depressive illness. The full-blown illness may be preceded by a prodromal phase with symptoms including social isolation or withdrawal, impairment in role functioning, peculiar behavior, impairment in personal hygiene, affect disturbances, thought disturbances manifested by vague, digressive, circumstantial, or metaphysical speech, bizarre ideation or magical thinking, and unusual perceptual experiences, which may not be diagnosable as clear hallucinations. Similar symptoms are seen in remission with or without treatment. The currently recognized subtypes follow.

*Rypins' Intensive Reviews: Psychiatry and Behavioral Medicine,* by Gordon H. Deckert. Lippincott-Raven Publishers, Philadelphia © 1997.

## Subtypes of Schizophrenia

### DISORGANIZED TYPE (HEBEPHRENIA)

In addition to the clinical picture outlined previously, this relatively uncommon type shows blunted, inappropriate, and especially silly affect. Systemized delusions are characteristically absent and speech is frequently incoherent. Prognosis tends to be poor.

### CATATONIC TYPE

Here the schizophrenia is determined by any of the following: catatonic stupor, catatonic negativism, catatonic rigidity or posturing, and catatonic excitement. Onset is often acute. Introjection is a common defense mechanism. Prognosis is relatively good.

### PARANOID TYPE

The most common of the differentiated schizophrenias, the paranoid type, is dominated by persecutory or grandiose delusions or hallucinations with persecutory or grandiose content. Projection is a prominent defense mechanism.

### UNDIFFERENTIATED TYPE

The category of *undifferentiated* is used when the criteria for schizophrenia are met, but none of the previous three differentiations is in evidence.

### RESIDUAL TYPE

The diagnosis of residual type is used when there has been the history of at least one previous episode of frank schizophrenia, but on the present occasion the clinical picture does not present prominent psychotic symptoms, although there is continuing evidence of illness.

## Incidence

Schizophrenia constitutes the largest group of severe behavioral disorders in our culture. About 1% to 3% of the population are affected. It is seen most commonly in lower socioeconomic groups, especially in areas of high mobility and social disorganization. One explanation for the prevalence in these groups is the "downward drift" hypothesis, which essentially states that schizophrenic patients move toward such a lower socioeconomic categorization. Onset is usually between 20 and 40 years of age, although it may be earlier. It is unusual for a first episode to appear after age 45 years. Long-term studies suggest that there is not a separate category of childhood schizophrenia, and that schizophrenia in childhood or adolescence simply represents the earlier appearance of schizophrenic illness.

## Etiology

The etiology of schizophrenia is unknown. There is evidence for both genetic and biochemical components. Various studies suggest left hemisphere dysfunction; dilated ventricles in a subgroup of patients; a high state of dopamine activity, especially with acute illness; and, conversely, a low state of dopamine activity in others, especially those with chronic illness. Psychodynamic formulations are many but currently focus on a disturbance of ego with an inability to differentiate between self and object and unusual sensitivity to sensory input. Psychoanalytic theory views the logic of schizophrenia as primary process thinking and sees similarities to the associative patterns present in dreams and in fantasies, especially those of imaginative children.

Two broad categories of schizophrenia have been proposed: **process** schizophrenia, a variety in which the illness begins at a younger age and progresses slowly, seemingly inevitably toward a final state of deterioration; and **reactive** schizophrenia, which begins temporally in relation to a traumatic event and is often of acute onset. The latter seemingly has a better prognosis. In fact, if a patient is hospitalized for less than 3 months with the first illness, the remission rate is at least 75%. If the patient has been hospitalized for over 2 years, the remission rate is approximately 1% to 2%.

## Treatment

Treatment is **empiric**. **Antipsychotic agents** are indicated. Hospitalization during the acute illness is often required. Although difficult to obtain, the development of a trusting doctor–patient relationship that can be maintained over time seems particularly important, whereby the physician, so to speak, becomes an auxiliary reality tester for the patient and helps the patient in a growing-up process. The absence of a familial or community support system seems to trigger exacerbation of illness and rehospitalization. Today, every schizophrenic patient should be given an adequate trial of pharmacologic treatment, usually one of the phenothiazines, although newer drugs with fewer side effects show promise.

# OTHER PSYCHOTIC DISORDERS

Some patients who are psychotic do not present with the full picture of schizophrenia, but show persistent persecutory delusions or delusions of jealousy with emotion and behavior appropriate to the content of these delusions, but without prominent hallucinations. There is no evidence of organic mental disorder, and the criteria for the manic–depressive syndrome are absent. If the illness is of at least 1 month's duration, the diagnosis of **delusional disorder** is made.

The diagnosis **schizophreniform disorder**, according to modern evidence and thought, is the appropriate appellation for patients who present with the symptoms of schizophrenia but in whom the illness, although lasting more than 2 weeks, has been present less than 6 months. Because many patients with such an acute illness recover without recurrence, labeling such people as schizophrenics is inappropriate. Frequently this disorder is in reaction to an acutely stressful life event. Patients with a borderline personality seem particularly subject to such responses.

Some patients seem to have a mixture of schizophrenia and a major affective disorder with symptoms such that neither diagnosis can clearly be made. For some clinicians, the diagnosis **schizoaffective disorder** is used. There is controversy as to whether such a category is warranted.

A **brief psychotic disorder** is characterized by psychotic symptoms of more than 1 day's duration but lasting less than a month, frequently in response to unusually severe stress.

# Chapter 6

# Mood (Affective) Disorders

The principal and characteristic feature of the affective disorders is a **disturbance of mood**, especially depression, but mania or hypomania, anxiety, and anger may be present as well. These patients may be psychotic.

## MAJOR AFFECTIVE DISORDERS

A **manic episode** is characterized by a distinct period of an elevated, expansive, or irritable mood. Duration is of at least 1 week. In addition to the **mood disturbance**, there are frequently several or more of the following: increased activity or physical restlessness; increased talkativeness; flight of ideas or at least the subjective experience that thoughts are racing; inflated self-esteem to the point of grandiosity; seemingly decreased need for sleep; distractability; and an excessive involvement in activities that have a high potential for painful consequences, such as buying sprees and sexual indiscretions. In some patients, this may be accompanied by **psychotic features**, that is, impairment in reality testing with delusions, hallucinations, or bizarre behavior. Many patients with a manic episode do not present with psychotic features.

A major depressive episode is characterized by **dysphoric mood** or **anhedonia** (loss of interest or pleasure in usual activities and pastimes). The patient may describe the mood as depressed, sad, down in the dumps, or irritable. A sense of helplessness and hopelessness is very common, as is guilt and such accompanying emotional states as anxiety and anger. These symptoms should be present nearly every day for a period of at least 2 weeks. They are accompanied by several of the following: poor appetite and significant weight loss or, in some patients, increased appetite with significant weight gain; insomnia or, in some patients, hypersomnia; psychomotor agitation or retardation; loss of interest in usual activities or decrease in sexual drive; loss of energy and a sense of fatigue; feelings of worthlessness and self-reproach with excessive or inappropriate guilt; complaints of diminished ability to think or concentrate; and recurring thoughts of death or suicidal ideation or a history of a suicide attempt.

There may be **psychotic features** with delusions and hallucinations. When the subjective experience of depression is particularly severe, when the depression seems worse in the morning and is often accompanied by early morning awakenings, psychomotor retardation or agitation, significant anorexia or weight loss, and profound guilt, the term **melancholia** is often used.

## Bipolar Disorder

Over time, patients with **bipolar disorder** (**manic–depressive** illness) cycle between the features of both manic and depressed episodes. In some people, depressive episodes predominate, and in others manic episodes predominate. In a smaller percentage, the episodes are intermixed, rapidly alternating every few days.

## Major Depression

Patients with **major depression (unipolar, endogenous)** meet the requirements of a major depressive episode as described earlier, but have never had a manic episode. They may or may not have a past history of a major depressive episode.

## Incidence

More than half of patients with bipolar disorders become ill before age 30 years. Unipolar onsets reach their peak in the fifth decade. Bipolar disorders are equally distributed in men and women. Manic episodes typically begin more suddenly than depressive episodes and may last from a few days to months, but tend to be briefer in duration than depressive episodes. In some patients, perhaps 20%, the course seems chronic. Epidemiologic evidence suggests that about 20% of women and 10% of men will have a depressive episode sometime in life, with hospitalization required in about 6% of women and 3% of men.

## Etiology

The precise etiology of these diseases is unknown. There is good evidence that the illness is familial, and for some there is clearly a genetic component, especially those with bipolar illness as well as a group of patients who have recurring unipolar depression. There is also evidence of a disturbance in those neurotransmitter systems based on the catecholamines. For some patients, recurring major depression seems to be related to specific identifiable stress. Some patients have a single major depression in their lifetime. Psychogenesis seems more prominent in the latter groups. Personality structure, to some degree, predicts treatment resistance and degree of recovery.

## Treatment

Depending on the severity of the illness, treatment may involve electroconvulsive therapy, drug therapy, or psychotherapy. Electroconvulsive therapy is particularly efficacious in a high percentage of patients with depression. Most clinicians use electroconvulsive therapy after an unsuccessful trial of drug intervention. Phenothiazines, especially haloperidol, may be initially useful in manic states. **Lithium**, however, is currently the treatment of choice in bipolar disease, especially to effect prevention of manic episodes. (However, other drugs have been and are being developed as well.) Although lithium may also be useful in the treatment of some patients with recurring unipolar depression, a full trial of an antidepressant drug is the treatment of choice for major depression. **Psychotherapy is extremely difficult** and is usually disappointing if there is the expectation of significant improvement in mood or energy level. However, studies do show that patients can achieve significant improvement in self-esteem and in interpersonal relationships. In addition, the relationship established with the physician facilitates psychopharmacologic intervention.

More recent studies indicate that maintenance therapy with antidepressant medications prevents recurrence and is indicated in patients with a past history of recurring major depressive episodes. Maintaining a relationship with a therapist facilitates recovery and also decreases the likelihood of recurrence.

# OTHER AFFECTIVE DISORDERS

## Cyclothymic Disorder (Cyclothymic Personality)

Some patients present with a history of numerous periods in which symptoms characteristic of both depressive and manic syndromes are present but are not of such severity to meet the criteria of either a major depressive or manic episode. These episodes are also separated by periods of normal mood that may last for months. Although some patients may proceed over time to frank bipolar illness, many do not, and these tend to be viewed by some as people in whom this personality disorder has developed in response to psychological factors, and by others as subclinical cases of bipolar disease.

## Dysthymic Disorders (Depressive Neurosis)

Current criteria for this diagnosis require at least a 2-year history of symptoms characteristic of a depressive syndrome but not of such severity to meet the criteria for a major depressive episode. There may be periods of normal mood lasting for a few days to a few weeks. There are clearly no psychotic features. This diagnostic entity is more common than bipolar or unipolar disease in primary care settings.

Although some patients benefit from antidepressant medication, many do not. In fact, some seem to become even worse. **Psychotherapy** is the usual mode of treatment. Careful studies evaluating the effectiveness of psychotherapy show distinct benefit compared with control groups, and in some studies psychotherapy alone shows better outcome than psychotherapy plus antidepressant medication.

Psychotherapy seems particularly helpful when the depression has been triggered by an identifiable life stress. The term **reactive depression** is often used in this instance. A careful study of these patients often suggests a vulnerability to certain kinds of stress, especially loss, through earlier life events and the elaboration of a particular character structure. **Introversion** is a common defense mechanism. Some patients' complaints, especially in primary care settings, are primarily somatic. Some clinicians see these patients as suffering from **depressive equivalent**. If treatment is focused only on the somatic complaints, improvement at best is only transitory; the underlying depression must be recognized and treated. Some patients with dysthymia experience a major depressive episode, and the term **double depression** is sometimes used here.

## Other Disorders Suggestive of Depression

Many, perhaps most, patients in ambulatory primary care settings whose complaints suggest depression do *not* fall into *any* of the previous diagnostic categories. Many patients who speak of themselves as depressed have experienced losses and are responding appropriately with grief; these patients are manifesting **uncomplicated bereavement**. Therapy facilitating the grief work is the physician's major responsibility.

Others are responding to an identifiable stressor, often a loss, in a maladaptive way, and the diagnosis **adjustment disorder with depressed mood** is appropriate. Here, again, psychotherapeutic intervention is indicated, and rarely psychopharmacologic intervention.

Finally, a number of physical conditions may be accompanied by depression, including carcinoma of the lung, carcinoma of the head of the pancreas, and myxedema. Certain drugs can precipitate a depressive syndrome (e.g., reserpine). The appropriate diagnosis in these instances is a **mood disorder due to the medical illness or the drug** in question, and such patients should be treated accordingly. Again, in older people, depression may mimic or accompany dementia.

Depression is one of the most common complaints bringing patients to physicians. Some studies indicate that it is *the* most common complaint. Other studies suggest anxiety, and still others, depending on the season, list upper respiratory complaints. A final reminder—depression should alert the physician to evaluate the risk for suicide.

# Chapter 7

# *Anxiety Syndromes*

This nosologic category and several that follow represent disturbances or disorders that previously have been called the psychoneuroses. "Neurotic," as used in this review, is not a pejorative term. It is descriptive. Whatever the etiology, it connotes a pattern of responses that is maladaptive. These disorders do not show gross disturbances of reality testing or severely antisocial behavior, and in the main are determined by environmental factors. The factors in part are in the present, consisting of those precipitating stresses that immediately precede an exacerbation of psychoneurotic symptoms. These factors also relate to the past, when environmental influences acting on the infant or the child produced a defect in personality development, leaving the person vulnerable to the later elaboration in adult life of neurotic patterns of response. To a degree, the childhood experience for all of us becomes the paradigm for all that follow. These predominantly learned responses are either adaptive or maladaptive, and they can be unlearned.

Key to understanding psychoneurosis is the concept of **conflict**, which may be partially conscious but is mainly unconscious. A person must be carefully evaluated to determine what in fact represents a significant conflict and, beyond that, a conflict related to a neurotic disorder. Conflict tends to develop around the issues of dependency, aggression, sexuality, or some mixture thereof. Subjective and objective evidence for emotions during the evaluation frequently suggests the nature of the conflict, especially those emotions experienced or displayed when discussing significant present situations reminiscent of past events, and those linked to the exacerbation of neurotic symptomatology. As the conflict becomes more conscious, and hence better understood, there is enhanced opportunity for change.

## PHOBIC DISORDERS

With phobic disorders, repression followed by isolation and displacement are characteristic defense mechanisms. In some patients, the maladaptive response evolves from those conflict issues typical of a child from age 3 through 6 years. Premorbidly, an avoidant or compulsive personality is common. Phobias have a higher prevalence rate than any other disease, including upper respiratory infections.

## Agoraphobia

These patients have a marked fear of and thus **avoid being in public places** from which there may be no immediate escape. They usually restrict their normal activities to the point that avoidance behavior dominates their life. To venture forth is to experience overwhelming, incapacitating anxiety. One group of patients has a history of **severe panic attacks**, whereas another group does not. In the group with panic attacks, the attacks often occur without evidence of there being a particular understandable situational stress related to a particular underlying conflict. The person's response to these panic attacks is to become increasingly phobic. Management of the panic attacks with preventive medication together with appropriately structured psychotherapy may be the treatment of choice for this particular group. In short, in one group the agoraphobia is primary and the anxiety is secondary; in the other, panic attacks are primary and the agoraphobia is secondary. Treatment is different for each group.

## Social Phobia

These patients experience a persistent, irrational fear of and a desire to avoid a situation in which they are exposed to possible scrutiny by others. The patient recognizes that the **fear is excessive or unreasonable,** but feels powerless to effect change. In some, this fear can become almost totally incapacitating.

## Specific (Simple) Phobia

Here, the irrational fear is of an object or a situation other than being away from home (agoraphobia) or anxiety regarding social situations (social phobia). Fear of animals, heights, and close spaces are examples. Again, the patient recognizes that the fear is excessive or unreasonable. Therapy may include dynamic psychotherapy, the technique of reciprocal inhibition, or behavioral therapy using some schedule for desensitization.

# ANXIETY DISORDERS

## Panic Disorder

With this disorder, the patient presents with a **history of distinct** panic attacks, which occur in the absence of a life-threatening situation or marked physical exertion, but are usually of rapid onset and of minutes' to hours' duration. The patient describes subjective awareness of severe anxiety, apprehension, or fear, and usually reports several or more physical symptoms that are in the category of the typical psychophysiologic manifestations of anxiety, such as dyspnea, palpitations, sweating, trembling, and so forth. These patients often appear in emergency rooms convinced they are in the throes of a life-threatening illness. Referral to a cardiologist is common. For a subgroup of patients, there is a family history. A genetic factor probably is present etiologically.

Management of the panic attacks requires **pharmacologic intervention**. Psychotherapy alone does not stop the attacks in this group of patients. On the other hand, not all patients with panic attacks have a panic disorder. With panic attacks, avoidant behavior often develops secondarily, as does anticipatory anxiety, the anxiety related to the fear of having another panic attack.

## Generalized Anxiety Disorder

Anxiety is an extraordinarily common complaint of patients in primary care ambulatory settings. This disorder is to be distinguished from normal fear of real, life-threatening situations or from an adjustment reaction manifested by anxiety. Certain illnesses mimic this disorder (e.g., hyperthyroidism, mitral valve prolapse syndrome, pheochromocytoma); however, these patients frequently describe their symptoms as being qualitatively different (e.g., they often describe their symptoms as feeling *as if* they were afraid).

### *Characteristics*

This disorder is characterized by the manifestations of anxiety, either consistently present or frequently recurring. The patient may report a subjective awareness of this anxiety, using such expressions as fear, afraid, apprehension, worry, and so forth; describe feeling constantly on the alert, dreading some unknown and unidentified danger or tragedy; or report various of the psychophysiologic manifestations of anxiety (e.g., sweating, feeling cold, clammy hands, lightheadedness, or a combination of these various groups of symptoms). Patients who report the physiologic manifestations of anxiety may deny feeling apprehensive, anxious, or fearful. Other patients who describe overwhelming fear and anxiety may not in fact look fearful or anxious to the physician (i.e., are **incongruent**).

Psychotherapeutic intervention is different for the different subgroups described. However, even when the patient feels anxious, reports the symptoms of anxiety, and appears anxious to the physician (i.e., is **congruent**), the patient rarely fully or even adequately understands the basis for the anxiety, or if he or she does link it to a particular situation or event, the linkage does not make sense to him or her.

**Repression** and **denial** are common **defense mechanisms**. Some authorities believe that the neurotic personality structure (often a histrionic personality) and the neurotic symptoms frequently date to those conflicts and issues typical of children 4 to 7 years of age.

**Psychopharmacologic agents**, if used, should be used judiciously, and then usually only for brief periods. Some form of psychotherapy ordinarily is the treatment of choice.

## Obsessive–Compulsive Disorder

Obsessions or compulsions become a significant source of distress to the degree that they interfere with social or role functioning. These patients are particularly distressed in knowing their symptoms are irrational. **Reaction formation**, **undoing**, and **overintellectualization** are typical **defense mechanisms**. The premorbid personality sometimes is a compulsive personality, which in many patients dates to particular responses to conflicts and issues of childhood typical of ages 1.5 to 3 years. Frequently the patient presents behaviorally as a clean, neat, overly polite person who speaks in a rather controlled and guarded fashion, but in others this is not the case. Although subjective awareness of anxiety and sadness may be present, there is typically an absence of evidence for anger. In fact, many patients either take pride in the infrequency of their experiencing anger or express considerable fear of it.

"Obsessive–compulsive disorder" and "compulsive personality" are not synonymous terms, and usually one does not relate to the other.

**Psychotherapy** is often the treatment of choice, but the course may be long and difficult. In some, this disorder is familial and a genetic factor is postulated etiologically. Studies implicate the serotonin neurotransmitter systems, and antiserotonin pharmacologic agents may reduce symptoms significantly.

## Posttraumatic Stress Disorder

Posttraumatic stress disorder merits a separate diagnostic category. In response to a specific recognizable stressor that would tend to evoke symptoms of distress in almost anyone, these patients continue to reexperience the trauma. This is manifest through either recurring dreams, or intrusive recollections of the event, or subjective sensations that the event is occurring again, triggered in association with an environmental or thought stimulus reminiscent of the trauma. Examples of typical stressors include accidents, combat, surgery, deaths, and the like. In addition, these patients may report a numbing of responsiveness to the external world manifest by markedly diminished interest in previously significant activities and subjective feelings of detachment or estrangement from significant others. There are frequently exaggerated startle responses, sleep disturbances, guilt about surviving when others have not, trouble concentrating, avoidance behavior toward activities that might trigger recollection of the event, and intensification of symptoms by exposure to events that symbolize the traumatic occurrence.

Some form of **psychotherapy** is the preferred treatment, together with **group therapy**. Prognosis is usually good with early intervention. If duration of symptoms is less than 3 months, the modifier **acute** is applied, if over 5 months the term **chronic** is used, and if onset is at least 6 months after the stressor, the specifier **with delayed onset** is used. (As I write this review, I am seeing patients with this disorder as a consequence of the Oklahoma City bombing, among survivors and rescuers alike, including some health professionals who rushed to the scene.)

# Chapter 8

# Somatoform Disorders

**Briquet's syndrome** is characterized by **multiple somatic complaints** not adequately explained by physical disorder, injury, or side effects of medication or drugs. These patients typically report that they have been sickly all or a good part of their lives. Complaints include symptoms that might fall into the conversion or pseudoneurologic category (e.g., loss of voice, double vision, muscle weakness, difficulty urinating), gastrointestinal symptoms (e.g., abdominal pain, nausea, bloating), female reproductive symptoms (e.g., painful menstruation, menstrual irregularity, severe vomiting through pregnancy), psychosexual symptoms (e.g., pain during intercourse, sexual indifference, lack of pleasure during intercourse), pain (e.g., in back, joints, extremities), and cardiopulmonary symptoms (e.g., shortness of breath, palpitations, dizziness). Current diagnostic criteria require at least a dozen of such symptoms and a history of several years' duration beginning before age 30 years.

There may be a **genetic disposition** to this disorder. There is often a family history of a similar syndrome, especially in female relatives, or antisocial behavior, especially in male relatives, or alcoholism. A history of multiple trials of medications without significant change in symptomatology is common. Pharmacotherapy seems to have little value. These patients are very resistant to treatment. This disorder should be distinguished from hypochondriasis.

Conversion disorders are characterized by an **involuntary psychogenic loss** or **disorder of function** often suggesting a physical illness. Symptoms typically are limited to impairment of motor or sensory functions (e.g., blindness, paresthesia, paralysis), but also may involve the autonomic system to a lesser degree. Symptoms characteristically begin and end suddenly. Often symbolic of an underlying conflict, the symptoms resolve, so to speak, the underlying dilemma. In psychodynamic terms, this is called the **primary gain**.

A **secondary gain** is often superimposed, such as avoiding some unpleasant activity, obtaining additional attention from significant others, avoiding responsibility, and so forth. Many patients give the impression of being naive, and some behave in a seductive fashion toward the examiner, or may seem strangely indifferent or aloof to their symptomatology (*la belle indifférence*), and yet under certain circumstances demonstrate poor emotional control.

These patients are frequently misdiagnosed as malingerers by the general medical profession. **Repression**, **denial**, and **dissociation** are common **defense mechanisms**. It is not unusual for a patient to have few if any memories reaching before age 6 years. A premorbid histrionic character is common, frequently with an underlying sexual conflict reminiscent of the oedipal conflict of ages 4 through 7 years.

**Psychotherapeutic intervention** may be dramatically successful, especially early in the course of the illness. **Hypnotherapy** may be especially helpful in some patients. If symptoms have been present for months or years, therapy becomes difficult. This is also the case when the disorder is superimposed over a physical illness.

# PAIN DISORDER

Here the predominant feature is **severe, prolonged pain**, often inconsistent with the anatomic distribution of the nerves, in the **absence of organic disease** or, when there is organic disease, the pain is grossly in excess of what would be expected from findings. Psychological factors are judged to be etiologically involved in the genesis of the pain. Some clinicians would see this syndrome as being a variation of a conversion disorder. Except for the symptom presentation, many of the statements made previously would apply to this category as well.

Some of these patients manifest a **chronic benign pain syndrome** (a term used by many authors). Patients with chronic depression constitute another major group. Many use multiple medications in large doses; some in fact are addicted. An intensive multidisciplinary treatment approach is required, with individual, group, and family therapy and a conservative approach toward pharmacotherapy. This syndrome is attracting increasing attention for many reasons, one of which is that a high percentage of resources from the health arena is devoted to this group of patients.

# HYPOCHONDRIASIS

The predominant disturbance here is an **unrealistic interpretation of physical signs** or **sensations** as abnormal, leading the patient to a preoccupation with the fear of or belief in having a serious disease, a disease that tends in the patient's view to go unrecognized by family and physicians. The malady causes considerable social and occupational impairment, tends to persist despite medical reassurance that no such disease exists, and often becomes the central theme around which the family is organized. In this manner, control and attention are obtained simultaneously. Patients, therefore, tend to have serious **conflicts** in the area of **dependency and aggression**. Considerable psychotherapeutic skill is needed in working with this group of patients.

# DISSOCIATIVE DISORDERS

Subgroups in this category include psychogenic amnesia, psychogenic fugue, multiple personality, and depersonalization disorder. All are predominantly psychogenic in origin.

## Amnesia

Amnesia refers to the sudden inability to recall important personal information that is too extensive to be explained by forgetfulness. A **fugue** is characterized by the assumption of a new identity by the patient, who often travels away from home or usual place of work and is unable to recall the past. During a fugue a patient may seem to behave normally to the casual observer.

## Multiple Personality

Multiple personality is defined as the existence within a given person of two or more distinct personalities, each of which predominates at a particular time. Many statements made about patient characteristics, etiology, and treatment under the Conversion Disorder section apply to this group as well. Patients with multiple personality usually have a very complex personality structure, and considerable psychotherapeutic skill is required for a successful outcome. They often have a history of severe and recurrent abuse as a child, either physical or sexual, or both. Frequently, that history becomes evident only during therapy. A recent term is **dissociative identity disorder**.

## Depersonalization Disorder

Patients with a depersonalization disorder respond to neurotic conflicts in such a manner that they experience parts of their bodies as not belonging to them or as greatly expanded or changed in size or shape, or they may experience themselves as unreal, phony, in a fog, and so forth. The experience is often **transient** and in response to a meaningful life event, but often is not recognized as such by the patient. When the condition is severe, patients may seem psychotic. Symptoms of derealization—that is, the sensation or feeling that the surround is strange or unreal—may or may not accompany the depersonalization. Depersonalization is also experienced with sleep deprivation, and by people under severe and prolonged stress (e.g., tortured prisoners of war).

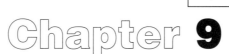

# Chapter 9

# Sexual and Gender Disorders

Current nosology categorizes psychosexual disorders into the **gender identity disorders**, including gender identity disorder of childhood and of adults (transsexualism); the **paraphilias**, including fetishism, frotteurism, transvestism, zoöphilia, pedophilia, exhibitionism, voyeurism, sexual masochism, sexual sadism, and transvestic fetishism; and the **sexual dysfunctions**. Egodystonic homosexuality is also considered a psychosexual disorder by some, although it has been dropped from *DSM-IV*. Egodystonia refers to the fact that the person is uncomfortable with and does not want a particular set of symptoms. In this instance, the patient wishes not to be a homosexual in terms of fantasy, sexual arousal, or overt behavior. Behaviors that are egosyntonic do not cause subjective distress, *per se*.

## SEXUAL DYSFUNCTIONS

More commonly, the disorders seen in medical practice are sexual dysfunctions. One category is **hypoactive sexual desire disorder**. Here, the patient reports a persistent and pervasive inhibition of sexual interest. Often the patient does not experience this as a source of personal distress; the report of distress comes from the partner. With a **sexual aversion disorder**, the patient experiences disgust with and avoidance of almost all sexual contact.

Next are **sexual arousal disorders**. Here, the patient reports sexual interest, but, for men, there is partial or complete failure to attain or maintain erection throughout the sexual act, and, for women, the partial or complete failure to attain or maintain the lubrication and swelling response of sexual excitement throughout the act. **Female orgasmic disorder** is a recurring and persistent pattern of delay or absence of orgasm, although there has been normal sexual excitement. **Male orgasmic disorder** is similarly defined.

**Premature ejaculation** refers to ejaculation occurring before the person wishes it because of an inability to bring reasonable voluntary control of ejaculation to the sexual act. Obviously the term "reasonable control" requires clinical judgment. This diagnosis is probably made too frequently by both physicians and patients. A patient may insist that he is a premature ejaculator, yet on careful inquiry the length of time or the number of sexual thrusts during intercourse is at or above average.

**Functional dyspareunia** refers to pain during intercourse of psychogenic origin. This diagnosis also is made too frequently. Discomfort may occur because the penis is inserted before the woman has reached the plateau phase; communication between partners usually solves this problem. Foreplay may take place with the patient exclusively on her back, and introital lubrication does not take place given the slant of the vagina; therefore, insertion is uncomfortable. In some women, with deep penetration, penile thrusting impinges on the cervix, causing pain; here a change in position during intercourse often effects a solution. For all these circumstances, educational counseling is indicated. Major psychogenic factors may not be playing a role.

**Functional vaginismus** refers to voluntary spasm of the musculature of the outer one third of the vagina, hindering or preventing insertion. In some patients, this is essentially a conversion reaction; in others, it has become a learned response. Psychotherapy is probably the treatment of choice for the former group, behavior therapy for the latter.

## Diagnosis

All of the diagnostic categories under "sexual dysfunction" are disturbances not caused exclusively by organic factors. Again, **psychogenic factors** predominate. Anxiety regarding the sexual act or hostility between partners is the typical psychodynamic picture. Commonly, symptoms may be present with one partner but not another, or historically symptoms may not be present before marriage but may appear after marriage (the reverse is just as frequent). In some instances an unresolved oedipal problem plays a dynamic role. In others, the symptoms seem to result from early life messages that the person was not to assume an adult sexual role or that the sexual act in some fashion was ugly or dirty.

When evaluating these patients, especially those in whom functional dyspareunia and inhibited orgasm are suspected, a careful medical workup including history and laboratory tests is indicated, because a number of medical conditions may first be manifest with one of these problems as the primary symptom. Penile erection studies are being used in this regard. Full erections take place during rapid eye movement sleep; if such are reported or demonstrated, erectile difficulties are most likely psychogenic in origin.

# Chapter 10

# Adjustment Disorders

DIAGNOSIS

The diagnosis of adjustment disorder should be used frequently, especially in primary care settings. These patients present with mental, emotional, or behavioral symptoms in response to a given life event, but the criteria for the diagnostic categories outlined in previous chapters are not met. However, there is evidence of a **maladaptive reaction to an identifiable social stressor** within 3 months of the onset of the stressor. The maladaptive nature of the reaction is indicated by impairment in social or occupational function or by symptoms that seem in excess of a normal or expected response to such a stressor. With this diagnosis, it is assumed that the symptoms would remit should the stressor cease, or a new level of adaptation be achieved should the stressor persist.

Depending on the predominant manifestation, the diagnosis of adjustment disorder is modified by one of the following self-explanatory phrases: with **anxious mood**, with **depressed mood**, with **mixed emotional features**, with **disturbance of conduct**, with **mixed disturbance of emotions and conduct**, with **work or academic inhibition**, with **withdrawal**, and, finally, with **atypical features**. These disorders are to be distinguished from normal fear, anger, or grief responses to the stresses of injury, frustration of real need, or loss, respectively.

TREATMENT

Most patients with adjustment disorders can be helped with **supportive** or **educational psychotherapy** or counseling. In general, neither pharmacotherapy nor referral for intensive psychotherapy are indicated. If a new level of adaptation does not occur or if symptoms persist or become worse, then the diagnosis of adjustment disorder no longer applies; the diagnosis should be changed and treatment strategies developed accordingly.

# Chapter 11

# Psychological Factors Affecting Physical Conditions

Psychologically meaningful environmental stimuli may be temporally related to the initiation or exacerbation of physical conditions, conditions that either have a demonstrable organic pathology or a known pathophysiologic process. An example of the latter would be tension headaches, and of the former, ulcerative colitis. A great number of patients fall into this category. The pathophysiology of such illness is increasingly well known and is not reviewed in detail here. Psychologically significant events or trains of events often linked to situations or events reminiscent of childhood or adolescence are interpreted in the cortex. Then, with involvement of the limbic system, the hypothalamic–pituitary–adrenal axis and the hypothalamic–autonomic nervous system axis trigger pathophysiologic responses or accentuate existing pathologic processes.

Many patients have difficulty understanding how psychological or social factors can contribute to their illness. A trusting relationship with their physician is of prime importance, as is skill in communicating this understanding. Even then, patients frequently do not recognize their conflict areas or areas of stress. In fact, in many instances, it is difficult for the clinician to determine these as well. A careful psychosocial history relative to the onset of the illness or the exacerbations or remissions in the illness may provide clues in this regard, as may the patient's use of "body language," that is, such figures of speech as "pain in the neck," "he makes me sick to my stomach," "it just breaks my heart."

Therapeutic intervention often requires the cooperation of a number of medical specialties. In addition to traditional medical management, psychotropic medication, behavioral modifying techniques, and psychotherapy may be used as well.

*Rypins' Intensive Reviews: Psychiatry and Behavioral Medicine,* by Gordon H. Deckert. Lippincott-Raven Publishers, Philadelphia © 1997.

# MAJOR ILLNESSES WITH PSYCHOLOGICAL FACTORS

The following represents a brief outline of the organ systems to which disorders of this category may apply.

## Skin Disorders

Psychological factors are prominent in patients with dermatitis factitia, trichotillomania, pruritus, and neurodermatitis, and may be significant with alopecia, urticaria, rosacea, psoriasis, herpes, and hyperhidrosis, as well as others.

## Musculoskeletal Disorders

**Musculoskeletal tension headache** is one of the most common symptoms of humankind. Similarly, pain involving skeletal musculature elsewhere, whether in the chest or back or in the extremities can result from underlying psychophysiologic mechanisms. Immunologic abnormalities seem significant in rheumatoid arthritis, but stress reactions acting through the hypothalamus can affect immune mechanisms. The common observation that some patients with **rheumatoid arthritis** have exacerbations of symptoms under emotional stress should not be ignored.

## Respiratory Disorders

The **hyperventilation syndrome** is the most common syndrome in this category. Frequently it is a manifestation of underlying anxiety. However, depressed patients may hyperventilate, and hyperventilation may be a learned response without there necessarily being an underlying psychodynamic conflict of major significance. Psychological factors also seem to play a role in some patients with bronchial asthma and some patients with vasomotor rhinitis.

## Cardiovascular Disorders

Some patients with an underlying anxiety syndrome or acute sensitivity to body sensations may become aware of their cardiac function and become alarmed at what is essentially normal tachycardia. Emotional factors may play a role in certain cardiac arrhythmias. The precise relation between anxiety syndromes and the mitral valve prolapse syndrome requires further study. Certain categories of patients with **hypertension**, when studied psychiatrically, present evidence for a psychological component in their etiology. Difficulty in handling hostile feelings, difficulty in being assertive, and the presence of obsessive–compulsive traits are not uncommon. The so-called "type A personality" has been reported as being particularly prone to angina and coronary artery disease. This personality is characterized by an excessive competitive drive, a chronic sense of time urgency, a tendency to overcommit to a series of responsibilities, achievement orientation, and an immersion in self-imposed deadlines. Emotional factors play a role in vasodepressor syncope. There is evidence that emotional factors may precipitate sudden death in certain patients.

## Gastrointestinal Disorders

In addition to anorexia nervosa and bulimia, already described, this category includes cardiospasm, nervous vomiting, diarrhea, and constipation. Psychogenic factors play a role in ulcerative colitis in certain patients. In patients with **peptic ulcer disease**, some psychiatric investigations have reported a basic conflict between passivity and aggressiveness. **Reaction formation** is a common defense mechanism. Some clinical investigations have estimated that about 80% of gastric hyperactivity and hyperacidity is related to life situations.

## Genitourinary Disorders

In addition to the various sexual dysfunctions already reviewed, psychological factors can play a role in a wide variety of disturbances of genital and urinary functions. In certain people, life conflict influences menstrual disorders, abortion, leukorrhea, urinary frequency, urgency, retention, and prostatitis. Perhaps most dramatic is the amenorrhea of false pregnancy (pseudocyesis), in which there are other signs of pregnancy including breast changes, weight gain, and abdominal distention. This syndrome is almost entirely psychogenic in origin.

## Endocrine Disorders

**Obesity** is defined as an increase in adipose tissue of 15% or more above the norm for a given height and age. Psychological responses to obesity are nearly universal, and in most patients, psychological factors play a role in etiology. Group therapy seems particularly helpful in the treatment of obesity. Therapy limited to reducing diets and drugs frequently fails or, if successful, tends, in the overwhelming number of instances, to be followed by weight gain. The course of diabetes mellitus, hyperthyroidism, and myxedema is affected by psychological factors, and some investigators attribute a role in disease onset to such factors.

# ETIOLOGY

In the somatoform and dissociative disorders, the symptom is frequently symbolic of the conflict, but this is not the case in this group of disorders. In general, the effort to identify a specific constellation of psychological conflicts and relate them to specific psychophysiologic disorders has not been successful. If there is a personality type **prone to psychosomatic disease**, it would be the **compulsive personality**. However, all people seem more vulnerable to stress in one organ system than another. **Genetic predisposition** and early developmental factors probably play a more significant role in organ selection than personality type or the category of conflict. With these patients in particular, the conceptual principle of individual response specificity is essential for diagnosis and management. What life situations and life events represent a psychological stress to a specific patient, or which long-term psychological conflicts in fact are significant to a psychophysiologic process must be determined on an individual basis. The process of evaluation outlined in Chapter 2 is helpful in this regard, as is the biopsychosocial model as a way of thinking.

# CONDITIONS NOT ATTRIBUTABLE TO A MENTAL DISORDER*

All people over a lifetime, regardless of diagnosis, are confronted with particular problems of one kind or another and frequently turn to their physicians for assistance. When the problem is not caused by a mental disorder, when it is not a feature of one of the diagnostic categories described earlier, this problem should be recognized without attaching a diagnosis of mental disorder. Common examples of such problems that may be a focus of attention or treatment are borderline intellectual functioning, adult antisocial behavior (e.g., manifest in some professional thieves, dealers of illegal substances), malingering, academic problems, occupational problems, uncomplicated bereavement (especially common in the practice of medicine), noncompliance with medical treatment, phase-of-life problem, marital problems, parent–child problems, and other interpersonal problems.

The nosologic classifications discussed in Chapters 3 through 11 are known in American psychiatry as **axis I** conditions. They typically are what brings the patient to the physician. They are the diseases in the classic sense, as well as the dis-eases, from a normal fear response, to schizophrenia, to appendicitis, and so on. In Chapter 12, we will turn to axis II, where attention is paid to diagnosing the person.

---

*The following two paragraphs are not part of this chapter; however, the information is necessary for the understanding of succeeding chapters.

Chapter **12**

# Personality Disorders

## CHARACTERISTICS OF PERSONALITY DISORDERS

Each of us has certain characteristic attitudes and reaction patterns in our relations to the world, to others, and to ourselves that make us unique. For each of us, the development of this character structure has a history. It begins in our early years and is elaborated over time. Although genetic influences play a role in temperament, there is little evidence, with some exceptions, that the various personality patterns have prominent genetic determinants *per se*. Much more prominent etiologically are all those events and situations of life to which a person responds over time with learned, acquired response patterns. Early mother–child interactions, familial example, discipline and teaching from significant others, peer relationships, unique personal experiences, cultural shaping, all contribute to our personalities. In summary, temperament interacts with environment and personality patterns emerge. When these ways of behaving become exaggerated, when behavior to some degree becomes stereotyped regardless of the external reality, the person then may be said to suffer from a character or personality disorder.

Frequently, people with such disorders experience little sense of distress over their personality. More often, others find them disturbing, or the person is distressed by the consequences of his or her character structure, often without awareness of how the character structure determined the very consequence he or she finds dis-easing. Each personality pattern disorder to some degree predicts that person's response to stress. Wise physicians include in their thinking the personality diagnosis of their patients. The management of appendicitis in a paranoid character is quite different than the management of appendicitis in a histrionic character. A paranoid character in delirium tends to behave differently from a histrionic character. The adjustment reactions of each to an identical stressful life event are different. Therapeutic intervention, therefore, in each instance varies.

When reviewing the following personality disorders, the reader would do well to ask a series of questions. If this personality disorder decompensated, would there be a tendency for the emergence of a particular mental disorder? If there were superimposed a delirium or a dementia, what would be the manifestations? If an anxiety disorder developed in this kind of person, what kind of stress, what kind of conflict would be most likely, and how would this effect management and treatment? How would this category of personality tend to respond to pregnancy, bronchoscopy, herniorrhaphy, diabetes mellitus, an intensive care unit, renal dialysis, paraplegia, loss of a job, malignancy in a young son, infidelity, divorce, death of a spouse, my characteristic way of opening an interview, my particular style of asking questions and giving suggestions? The list is almost endless, and lies at the heart of behavioral medicine.

Any nosology of personality disorders would be somewhat arbitrary. Many people show features of more than one category. Even within categories, the principle of individual response specificity still holds. Nonetheless, even when the personality pattern of a given patient does not warrant the label of a disorder, physicians limit their therapeutic potential if they fail habitually to diagnose the personality traits of their patients.

# CLUSTER A DISORDERS

The following group of disorders (known as Cluster A disorders in *DSM-IV*) tends to show greater psychopathology than those that follow, use more primitive defense mechanisms, and with decompensation under stress move toward more serious categories of mental illness.

## Schizotypal Personality Disorder

Although not meeting the criteria for schizophrenia, this personality type, as the name implies, has certain features of that illness. There tend to be magical thinking, ideas of reference, recurrent illusions, depersonalization not associated with manifest anxiety, and paranoid ideation. There is usually evidence for social isolation and undue social anxiety or hypersensitivity to real or imagined criticism. Speech is often odd, vague, circumstantial, or metaphoric, but without loosening of association or incoherence. There is inadequate rapport in face-to-face interaction with others. In addition, schizophrenia is commonly present in the extended family. These patients seem to have introjected a **semicrazy world**.

## Paranoid Personality Disorder

People of this type show a propensity for using **projection as a defense mechanism**. They demonstrate pervasive, unwarranted suspiciousness and mistrust of people. Hence, they are hypervigilant, expect trickery, are guarded or secretive, question the loyalty of others, tend to avoid accepting blame even when blame is warranted, look for hidden motives in the behavior of others, and often show unusual jealousy. They are often hypersensitive, tending to take offense quickly. They show restricted affectivity, appearing to be cold or unemotional, often taking pride in being, in their view, objective or rational. They often lack a sense of humor, and frequently there is an absence of soft, tender, sentimental feelings. In short, these people have been taught to **distrust the world**, to see conspiracies.

## Schizoid Personality Disorder

This type of personality is characterized by emotional coldness or aloofness, or absence of tender feelings toward others, and by relative indifference to praise or criticism or to the feelings of others. They tend to have very few if any close friends but may be very attached to animals. They may have outstanding academic records, having spent hours alone, studying. As adolescents they tend to be seen as shy and withdrawn. They give the appearance of being quiet loners. In contrast to the schizotypal personality disorders, there are, however, no major eccentricities in speech, behavior, or thought. In short, these people have been taught to **expect hurt** from the world but defend themselves by becoming **indifferent** to it.

# CLUSTER B DISORDERS

The following group of disorders (known as Cluster B in *DSM-IV*) tends to show less psychopathology than those in Cluster A, but more than those that follow.

## Antisocial Personality Disorder

Several of the following features are found in the history of these patients with onset **before age 15 years**: truancy, expulsion or suspension from school, behavioral delinquency, running away from home, persistent lying, casual sexual intercourse, repeated drunkenness or substance abuse, thefts or vandalism, poor school performance, chronic violation of rules at home, or initiation of fights.

**After age 18 years**, the disorder manifests as follows: an inability to sustain consistent work behavior, an inability to function in a consistent way as a responsible parent, failure to accept social norms with respect to lawful behavior, an inability to maintain enduring attachments to a sexual partner, irritability and aggressiveness as indicated by repeated physical fights or assaults, which may include spouse or child beating, failure to honor financial obligations with repeated defaulting on debts, failure to provide child support, failure to plan ahead, impulsive traveling from place to place without a clear goal in mind, disregard for the truth as indicated by lying, using aliases, and "conning" others, and recklessness.

Current diagnostic criteria require that such a behavioral pattern be present for at least 5 years without any intervening period in which the syndrome is absent. These people constitute a major social problem, consuming a considerable percentage of the human and fiscal resources of law enforcement, social service, and health agencies.

This disorder stands alone in this category in there being convincing data suggesting a major **genetic factor** in etiology. Early psychological factors also play a role. Particularly striking is the finding of a parental disciplinary pattern that is demanding, inflexible, and punitive one moment and permissive and nonpunitive the next. In short, these people behave as if they have **failed to incorporate any system of values**; hence, they are often described as **without conscience**.

## Borderline Personality Disorder

These people show many of the following characteristics. First, there tends to be impulsiveness in areas that are potentially self-damaging, for example, spending, sex, gambling, shoplifting, overeating, or physically self-damaging acts such as recurring accidents, self-mutilation, or suicide attempts. Drug or alcohol abuse is common. Second, there tends to be a pattern of unstable or intense personal relationships. Third, there is often inappropriate intense anger or lack of control in the expression of anger. Identity disturbances are commonly manifest by uncertainty over such issues as choice of friends, values, loyalties, or career. In short, there is considerable **difficulty with self-image**.

Next, there frequently is affective instability with marked shifts from normal mood to depression or irritability, usually lasting several hours but rarely for more than a few days, with a return to normal mood. They tend to be intolerant of being alone and experience chronic feelings of emptiness or boredom. For periods of time they seem to block out incoming stimuli, but on the other occasions seem exquisitely sensitive to it. Certain of these people under stress manifest "micropsychotic" episodes. During such episodes, the diagnosis of schizophreniform reaction may be appropriate.

Many physicians find these patients particularly difficult to understand or treat. They seem neither psychotic nor neurotic, or simultaneously both, but also normal from moment to moment. Although there is no convincing evidence to date for a genetic determinant for this disorder, the possibility of central nervous system dysfunction secondary to maturational lag or early developmental trauma is frequently raised by clinical investigators. These people behave as if they do not know who they are; they have a **chameleon quality**.

## Narcissistic Personality Disorder

Narcissists seem to possess a grandiose sense of self-importance or uniqueness and often are preoccupied with fantasies of unlimited success, power, brilliance, or beauty. There may be a quality of exhibitionism, that is, a requirement for attention. They may show cool indifference or marked feelings of rage, shame, or humiliation in response to criticism by others. Interpersonally, they tend to operate from the posture of entitlement, that is, the expectation of special favors from others without assuming reciprocity. There tends to be, therefore, **interpersonal exploitiveness**. They lack empathy and tend to relate to others by alternating between the extremes of overidealization and devaluation. Having never received or having received without the expectation of reciprocity, psychologically they seem like young children who simply **expect the world to revolve about them**; they would be quick to take umbrage with this description.

## Histrionic Personality Disorder

These people demonstrate behavior that is overly dramatic, reactive, and intensely expressed. This may be manifest by some of the following characteristics: self-dramatization with exaggerated expression of emotions, drawing of attention to self, a craving for activity and excitement, and overreaction to minor events, including irrational angry outbursts or tantrums. In addition, there are disturbances in interpersonal relationships. Often they are perceived by others as shallow and lacking in genuineness even if superficially charming, as egocentric, self-indulgent, vain and demanding, or sometimes as dependent and helpless, seeking constant reassurance. They demonstrate considerable denial and repression and at an unconscious level often sexualize their relationships with others, yet find sexual experience incomplete, unrewarding, or unsatisfying. These people psychologically seem stuck, fixated in the role of staying little boys or little girls.

# CLUSTER C DISORDERS

This last group of disorders (known as Cluster C disorders in *DSM-IV*) with decompensation tends to move toward less serious categories of mental illness than do those that precede it. This is a general statement, and not applicable in all instances. Further, the hierarchy is ordered with the assumption that "serious" refers to the more psychotic end of the spectrum of mental illness and "less serious" to the more neurotic. There would be those clinicians who would argue, quite appropriately, that this does not necessarily indicate less psychopathology.

## Dependent Personality Disorder

These people lack self-confidence and see themselves as **helpless** or **stupid**. They tend to subordinate their own needs to those of people on whom they depend. Their passivity allows others to assume responsibility for major areas of their life because of their inability to function independently. Because they seem so obedient and compliant, they are sometimes viewed by physicians as being "good" patients. Nonetheless, there is a tendency, so that they can maintain their dependency, for them to stay "sick" in one fashion or another. They can feel literally devastated with the loss of those on whom they depend—parent, spouse, employer, son, daughter, or physician. They have been taught that they cannot or should not function in the world as independent beings.

## Compulsive Personality Disorder

These people tend to be preoccupied with details, rules, order, organization, schedules, and lists. They often give themselves or are given the appellation of **perfectionist**. The perfectionist is one who attends to details and fails to grasp the larger picture. The compulsive personality frequently is unduly conventional or formal; has restricted ability to express warm and tender emotions; is unaware of feelings of anger even though the anger may be communicated to others nonverbally, or, if aware of anger, places premium on control of expression; and may be devoted almost excessively to work or studies to the exclusion of pleasure or interpersonal relationships. They tend to insist that others submit to their particular ways of doing things and seemingly are unaware of the feelings elicited in others by this behavior. Nonetheless, quite often they are indecisive, that is, decision making is postponed, avoided, or protracted from inordinate fear of making a mistake. In response, they adopt rules, principles, and belief systems that they automatically impose on themselves or on others in an arbitrary, unthinking fashion even when the situation does not particularly warrant that approach or response. They **lack flexibility**. Intellectualization, rationalization, compartmentalization, and reaction formation are typical defense mechanisms. In short, these people psychologically seem fixated on that stage of life where great emphasis is placed on "doing things right" at the risk of punishment, shame, withdrawal of love, or rejection.

## Avoidant Personality Disorder

This pattern of personality is characterized by hypersensitivity to rejection, an unwillingness to enter into relationships unless given strong guarantees of uncritical acceptance, social withdrawal, a desire for affection, and usually extremely low self-esteem. They avoid confrontation. They often appear to be afraid of success, but underneath desperately seek it. Outwardly they may behave in a manner similar to the schizoid, but these people are not indifferent to the world—they are **afraid of the world's shame and ridicule**.

## Mixed Personality Disorder

The **most common** disorder, however, is none of the previous. It is mixed personality disorder. Many people have features of more than one of those previously discussed, but do not meet the full criteria for a specific one. Even so, there is clinical evidence for distress or impairment of functioning.

One characteristic of normal, nonneurotic people is a personality structure that is not stuck or fixated into a particular pattern; hence, they demonstrate flexibility and adaptability. These people, sometimes called **genital characters**, may show features of any or all of the previous personality disorders. But, none of the above patterns predominates or endures when such behavior becomes maladaptive to a given situation. There are those who would insist that no one is normal, that everybody is neurotic or has some kind of neurotic personality disorder. However, this is simply not true.

It is estimated that about 20% to 30% of the adult population are genital characters, and another 20% to 30% might be viewed as near-genital characters. The concept of integration of certain features within a personality is useful when working with patients who are genital characters. It is useful to think in such terms as "a genital character with integrated compulsive features" or "a genital character with integrated histrionic features," and so forth. Genital characters not only **know who they are**, they **know from whence they cometh**; they recognize and enjoy their talents; they know their vulnerabilities. In summary, genital characters work effectively, love adequately, and play re-creatively.

A final comment: a competent patient-centered clinical practice *requires* diagnosis of the patient. This chapter has pointed the way.

# Chapter **13**

# *Prevention*

From within the health professions and from without, the growing emphasis on prevention derives from multiple factors: the realization that in most domains of medicine there seems to be almost no limit to the possible growth of treatment programs, the dramatically rising costs of medical care, and a genuine interest in the prevention of disability and suffering. Once again, note the leading actual causes of death in the United States in 1990 in Table 2-1. The predominant factor for most is behavior. This chapter considers the prevention of smoking, obesity, and alcohol abuse, and behavioral and emotional disorders in children, as examples. There is considerable evidence to suggest that successful techniques for prevention in these areas would have considerable impact on the incidence of a wide variety of diseases. The focus of behavioral medicine in this domain centers around a population-based clinical practice.

## ABSTINENCE

Abstinence can be achieved among heroin addicts, alcohol abusers, and smokers. For those who successfully maintain their abstinence, decreased incidence of certain illnesses has been documented. However, the relapse rates for these three addictions follow essentially a similar curve. After achieving abstinence, at 3 months only 40% remain abstainers, and after 12 months the figure falls to approximately 20%. A similar pattern holds for obesity. Programs for prevention too often are judged only in terms of immediate rates.

## Obesity

Initial reports on the use of **behavior therapy** compared with conventional programs for weight reduction were impressive, with behavior therapy programs outperforming the other approaches by impressive margins. However, with long-range studies, the overly optimistic expectations in this field have turned to disillusionment and pessimism, at least for some. Obesity after all is a life-style disorder; to effect the maintenance of weight reduction requires a life-style change. Some programs devoted to prevention have failed to confront the complexity of the problem and the repeatedly demonstrated difficulty in effecting major and enduring change in human behavior.

## Smoking

Another example is smoking. When smoking behavior is analyzed, it would appear that the main purpose in smoking technique is to get nicotine into the blood and particularly into the brain as quickly as possible. There is evidence that there has been a decrease in tobacco smoking in the United States. This has been attributed in part to a large-scale national education effort. However, the incidence of tobacco smoking has increased among adolescents in recent years in spite of this educational effort, especially among girls. Also, if one considers the increasing incidence of marijuana smoking in segments of the population, it is highly questionable whether in fact there has been an overall decreased incidence of smoking, *per se*. The proportion of people 18 to 25 years of age who have used marijuana has increased from 4% to 68% since 1962.

## Alcohol Abuse

The primary prevention of alcohol abuse poses similar problems. Alcohol education programs have been developed in schools. Studies of these programs suggest that students do make significant gains in their knowledge about alcohol, but changes in attitude and behavior do not necessarily follow. Actually, broader sociologic techniques may be more effective. For example, it is fairly clear from a variety of studies that those states that have lowered the legal drinking age have seen an increase in traffic accidents and fatalities and an increase in the number of young drinkers in treatment for alcoholism. Some studies suggest that the number of alcohol distribution outlets can be correlated to rates of consumption and of alcoholism.

## TECHNIQUES FOR PREVENTION

Other techniques for prevention have been developed to involve the population at risk more directly; an example is an instrument that asks the person to characterize his or her life-style. Then, using that data, they determine the likelihood of their succumbing to various diseases, given that life-style. Whether this approach effects change remains to be researched. The effect of a book on self-health care distributed to 460 families in a prepaid health plan has been reported. At 6- and 12-month study periods, there was no significant effect on the number of physician visits made, even though it was determined that half of the families read most of the book and a third used it specifically for a particular medical problem. All in all, in these areas it is clear that prevention on a large scale is a complex problem. Some have concluded that there has been more rhetoric regarding prevention than programs that have been demonstrated to work. Others point to studies showing some success, and argue that this is too pessimistic a view.

Various studies suggest that children born into a wanted and nurturing environment tend to receive good parenting and tend to have fewer behavioral and emotional problems in childhood. By inference, this group may show a lower incidence of mental illness as adults. But actually to effect an increase in the likelihood of children being born into such settings is difficult. In fact, the number of unwanted pregnancies, especially among teenagers, has increased, as has the number of teenagers keeping their babies. Sex education and abortion issues tend to generate very strong opinions. Current trends in the United States do *not* suggest a decrease in the number of unwanted children born into our population. Programs more narrowly focused and community based, however, show promise.

Depressed mothers are poor parents to infants. Programs to prevent depression in that population at high risk during the first 6 months postpartum are being developed. Their degree of success remains to be seen.

Some observers have suggested, rather caustically, that society will know when the medical profession takes prevention seriously when we see effective stress reduction programs in medical schools and in health science centers for the health professionals and the staff who work in such institutions.

# Chapter 14

# Treatment of Mental Illness

## THE PHYSICAL THERAPIES

### Electroconvulsive Therapy

The most common of the physical therapies in psychiatry is **electroconvulsive therapy** (ECT; or electroshock therapy). Although many theories have been postulated, the mode of action of this treatment is not certain. Empirically, there is no question that treatment produces remission in a high percentage of patients with severe depression. **Major depression** is almost a universally accepted indication for ECT, especially when the depression has not responded to pharmacotherapy or when the risk of suicide is high. On some occasions, patients with manic episodes also are treated with this modality. Patients with schizophrenia or with severe psychoneurosis are also sometimes treated in this manner, but indications here are controversial.

Many patients and their families approach ECT with some anxiety. When they understand the risks and benefits, the nature of the procedure, and especially when they have the opportunity to correct the distortions that many of them carry from portrayals in the media, this anxiety abates.

Historically, treatment was instituted by applying an alternating current through electrodes placed bitemporally, but considerable variations of technique have been introduced, including electrode placement at other sites, changes in the way the current is administered or in the properties of the current, and use of unidirectional currents and unilateral treatments. The advantages of the various methods are still primarily a matter of opinion; however, seizures, confusion, and memory loss are not necessarily required for therapeutic success. Treatments are typically given three times a week, up to 8 to 14 in a series. EEG changes occur almost universally, with slowing in all leads, becoming maximal after 10 to 12 treatments and disappearing in most cases within a few weeks.

*Complications*

The most common complication of ECT is an **induced cognitive disorder** with confusion and blurring of memory. This clears spontaneously. With modern techniques, the procedure has become exceedingly safe. There is certainly much less risk to the patient than the risk of suicide with unrelenting depression. Fractures and dislocations, especially compression fractures of the spine, have been considerably reduced with the use of muscle relaxants or subconvulsive therapy. Personnel must be prepared to deal with an occasional respiratory arrest or cardiac arrest. There would seem to be very few if any absolute contraindications, but special consideration should be given to patients who are pregnant or who have bone and joint disease, an aortic aneurysm, coronary artery disease, a recent myocardial infarction, a retinal detachment, a brain tumor, or increased intracranial pressure.

## Other Therapies

With the widespread use of **tranquilizing medications**, psychosurgery is now mainly of historic interest. Its most frequent application is in cases of intractable pain or focal seizures. **Light therapy** is indicated for a seasonal affective disorder, a type of major depressive episode.

## PHARMACOTHERAPY

Although the treatment of the mentally ill by means of drugs is not new, there has certainly been a renewed interest, even excitement, regarding drug therapy in the last several decades. The era of psychopharmacology came into being with the synthesis of chlorpromazine by Laborit in 1951. **Psychopharmacotherapy** aims at achieving better control of symptoms. It does not cure patients in the usual sense of the word. Medication must be prescribed on an individual basis with thorough knowledge of the patient's condition, a knowledge of the patient's reaction to the drug in question, and with a clear view of the therapeutic goal in mind. Compliance and outcome are enhanced when the patient participates in the decision, understands the expected outcome, and is prepared for possible adverse effects. There are many drugs used in the practice of psychological medicine. What follows is a brief and cursory review.

## Antipsychotic Agents (Major Tranquilizers, Neuroleptics, Ataractics)

Like the barbiturates, these agents have a **quieting** or **calming effect**, but unlike the older hypnotic agents, this occurs without producing marked drowsiness. Subcortical sites of action are more prominent than cortical effects. In general, these drugs cause accumulation of the O-methylated metabolites of dopamine and norepinephrine within the brain, suggesting that they block these brain receptor sites. The highest concentrations of these receptors are in the hypothalamus, the basal ganglia, the thalamus, the hippocampus, and the septum.

In addition to an antipsychotic effect, these drugs have an **antiemetic** effect. They also can result in **extrapyramidal symptoms** such as pseudoparkinsonism, akathisia (motor restlessness), dyskinesia, and torsion spasms. Some of these effects may be controlled by synthetic anticholinergic agents (e.g., benztropine mesylate, trihexyphenidyl hydrochloride). Of particular concern is **tardive dyskinesia**, which has a chronic course and usually appears after prolonged administration of such agents, with the symptoms often exaggerated when the drug is withdrawn. The dyskinesia is characterized by Parkinson-type activity of a choreiform character especially involving the tongue and the mouth. Other adverse effects include gynecomastia, heat intolerance (especially with chlorpromazine), pigmentation of the exposed areas of the skin, retinal pigmentation (especially with thioridazine), jaundice of the cholestatic type on occasion, and, less commonly, dermatitis and various blood dyscrasias. A neuroleptic malignant syndrome with cardinal features of elevated temperature and muscle rigidity can be a life-threatening complication. These drugs enhance the effects of central depressants such as barbiturates and alcohol.

This class of drugs is most useful with **schizophrenic disorders** and other **psychoses**. They also are used to help control the agitated or the hyperactive states of mania and the organic brain disorders. Some patients, in particular, respond with a marked decrease in the intensity of delusions and hallucinations. **Table 14-1** provides examples of the current six categories of antipsychotic agents, with the generic name followed by the trade name and the daily dose range. Newer agents (e.g., clozapine and risperidone) have been reported to be effective in patients who have had unsatisfactory responses to other classes of drugs, and to have fewer adverse effects in some instances.

## Antianxiety Agents (Anxiolytics, Minor Tranquilizers)

Antianxiety agents are used primarily to control the tension and anxiety seen in patients with **anxiety disorders** and in patients with **depression accompanied by agitation**. They have essentially replaced the use of barbiturates and sedatives in this regard. They have become one of the most commonly prescribed group of medications in the United States in all categories, psychiatric or otherwise, are subject to considerable abuse, and can become addictive. They are frequently used in suicide attempts. It is increasingly evident that caution should be used in prescribing these medications

**TABLE 14-1.**

**Psychopharmacologic Agents**

| Class | Generic Name | Brand Name | Daily Dosage (mg) |
|---|---|---|---|
| **Antipsychotic Agents** | | | |
| Phenothiazines | | | |
|   Aliphatic | Chlorpromazine | Thorazine | 50–1000 |
|   Piperidine | Thioridazine | Mellaril | 50–800 |
|   Piperazine | Fluphenazine | Prolixin | 1–20 |
| Thioxanthenes | Thiothixene | Navane | 5–60 |
| Butyrophenone | Haloperidol | Haldol | 1–100 |
| Dibenzoxazepine | Loxapine | Loxitane | 20–250 |
| | Clozapine | Clozaril | 50–900 |
| Dihydroindolone | Molindone | Lidone | 20–200 |
| Benzisoxazole | Risperidone | Risperdal | 4–6 |
| **Antianxiety Agents** | | | |
| Benzodiazepines | Alprazolam | Xanax | 0.5–6 |
| | Chlordiazepoxide | Librium | 15–100 |
| | Diazepam | Valium | 4–40 |
| | Oxazepam | Serax | 30–120 |
| Azaspirodecanedione | Buspirone | Buspar | 15–30 |
| Antihistamines | Hydroxyzine | Atarax | 50–400 |
| Carbonates | Meprobamate | Equanil | 200–1200 |
| **Antimanic Agents** | Lithium carbonate | Eskalith | 1200–1800 |
| **Antidepressants** | | | |
| Unicyclic | Bupropion | Wellbutrin | 100–300 |
| Tricyclics | Imipramine | Tofranil | 75–300 |
| | Nortriptyline | Aventyl | 75–150 |
| | Desipramine | Norpramin | 75–200 |
| | Amitriptyline | Elavil | 75–300 |
| | Doxepin | Sinequan | 75–300 |
| Tetracyclic | Maprotiline | Ludiomil | 150–225 |
| Monoamine oxidase inhibitors | Phenelzine sulfate | Nardil | 60–90 |
| | Tranylcypromine sulfate | Parnate | 10–30 |
| Serotonin reuptake inhibitors | Fluoxetine | Prozac | 10–80 |
| | Sertraline | | 50–200 |
| | Paroxitine | | 10–50 |

for more than short periods of time, but, given that caveat and with careful monitoring, they can be quite helpful. Short-acting and longer-acting agents each have their indication with particular groups of patients. Table 14-1 gives common examples of these agents.

Perhaps the most serious adverse effect of these agents is that long-term use tends to support the patient's tendency to avoid facing his or her psychological problems and effecting more appropriate solutions. In addition, when dosage is decreased or the drug is discontinued, withdrawal symptoms can be mistaken for heightened anxiety by the patient or the physician alike. The drugs produce mild sedation without major impairment of psychomotor performance. Drowsiness is perhaps the most common side effect. Patients should be warned about any activity involving skilled motor coordination, such as driving a car. These drugs have synergistic effects with alcohol and other sedatives, and patients should be forewarned. Other effects include dizziness, headache, dry mouth, and on occasion paradoxic hyperactivity, or rage reactions. Less common are hematologic, allergic, renal, and hepatic reactions.

β-Blockers (e.g., propranolol and atenolol), although not anxiolytic agents as such, do decrease peripheral symptoms. They can be useful in particular for patients who are especially reactive to such symptoms.

The **treatment of panic disorder** deserves special discussion. Prevention of panic attacks is critical. Preferred treatment is with a **tricyclic antidepressant** (e.g., imipramine), which has an inhibiting effect presumably at the level of the locus ceruleus. Alprazolam is also effective, but has risk for dependence. Whereas antianxiety agents as a class do not prevent attacks, imipramine and other tricyclic antidepressants do not dampen anticipatory anxiety, *per se*.

## Sedatives and Hypnotics

These drugs are used less and less in the practice of psychological medicine, but are still prescribed for **nighttime insomnia** and **severe daytime anxiety**. The antianxiety agents or even certain of the phenothiazines are probably better drugs of choice for severe daytime anxiety. After 2 to 3 days, the nighttime sedative effect begins to abate. In sleep laboratories, sedatives can be shown almost universally to have a disrupting effect on the sleep cycle. Earlier reports suggested there might be an exception to the latter statement, namely, flurazepam, but more recent studies raise questions regarding its disruption of the sleep cycle as well.

As an adjunct to certain phases of psychotherapy, short-acting barbiturates are used to induce a state of light narcosis (narcotherapy). It appears that all sedative–hypnotic preparations are potentially addicting.

## Central Nervous System Stimulants

There are perhaps only two indications for use of this class of drugs in the modern practice of psychological medicine. One is in the management of **hyperkinetic children**, where methylphenidate and pemoline are widely used. Methylphenidate and other amphetamines are also useful in the treatment of **narcolepsy**.

## Antimanic Agents: Lithium

**Lithium carbonate** is considered to be the standard antimanic drug for use in **bipolar disease**. Because it requires 7 to 10 days to achieve a threshold level in body tissues, acute episodes are usually managed initially with antipsychotic agents (e.g., haloperidol) until the lithium can begin to take effect. Long-term maintenance on lithium of patients with manic attacks is reported to prevent the recurrence of such attacks in 50% to 80% of patients. There is controversy as to whether lithium is effective in preventing recurring episodes of depression.

### Compliance

Compliance is a particular problem. Some patients "enjoy" their hypomania or carry with them the illusion, if not a grandiose delusion, that they are especially productive or creative in such a state. Also, lithium can bring a sense of "dullness" to the patient's experience. They frequently have difficulty in describing the effect. This reminds some patients of the early symptoms of depression, which they fear more than mania. This dullness usually abates over 6 to 12 months. Regular visits, repeated assurances, and an effective physician–patient relationship, as always, enhance compliance and outcome.

### Maintenance

Use of lithium requires the monitoring of blood levels. A therapeutic serum level of 0.5 to 1.5 mEq/L is usually in the therapeutic range. Because lithium competes with the sodium ion, it is not surprising that it is contraindicated in patients with renal, hepatic, or heart disease. With long-term administration, asymptomatic thyroid enlargement can occur. Most common side effects are polyuria, polydipsia, and a fine hand tremor. These tend to be transient in most patients. The range between a therapeutic level and toxicity is relatively narrow. As more toxic levels are reached, there is progressively the appearance of nausea and diarrhea, malaise, vomiting, muscle weakness, ataxia, abdominal pain, slurred speech, nystagmus, fasciculations, choreoathetoid movements, convulsions, circulatory failure, stupor, coma, and death. Extreme toxic effects have been reported at levels above 2.5 mEq/L.

In those patients who do not respond to lithium, anticonvulsants (e.g., carbamazepine) are sometimes effective.

## Antidepressants

As a group, antidepressants elevate mood, enhance mental alertness, improve sleep and appetite patterns, increase physical activity, reduce morbid preoccupations, and lower the risk of suicide in patients with depression. **Tricyclics** act by inhibiting the reuptake of norepinephrine and serotonin by the neuronal terminals.

**Monoamine oxidase (MAO) inhibitors** block intracellular metabolism of biogenic amines, resulting in an increased amine concentration at the terminals. Imipramine, nortriptyline, and desipramine seem to have more effect on norepinephrine systems, whereas amitriptyline and doxepin have a greater impact on serotonin. Patients who may not respond to one class of tricyclics may respond to another. All these compounds require 1 to 3 weeks before there is symptomatic response. **Serotonin reuptake inhibitors** (SRIs) are being used with increasing frequency. Table 14-1 provides some examples of these agents.

### Adverse Effects of Tricyclics

Tricyclics can aggravate the symptoms of schizophrenia and may convert depression into mania. **Adverse effects** include dry mouth, constipation, hyperhidrosis, and blurred vision. Weight gain has also been reported; less frequently, tachycardia, anorexia, increased ocular tension, urinary retention, and orthostatic hypertension.

### Maintenance with Monoamine Oxidase Inhibitors

MAO inhibitors are less effective than tricyclics and are usually used only after failure with tricyclics or ECT. Careful monitoring is needed because adverse reactions can be serious. These drugs should not be administered to patients taking other sympathomimetic compounds, often present in cold remedies and decongestants. Foods with high tyramine content should be avoided because hypertensive crisis may be precipitated. Subarachnoid hemorrhage has been reported. Other adverse reactions include orthostatic hypotension, dizziness, headache, cardiac arrhythmias, fatigue, dryness of mouth, blurred vision, and constipation.

Classes of antidepressants other than tricyclics have been introduced, such as buproprin and the SRIs. Whether they are more effective is not clear. Some seem to have fewer or less bothersome side effects.

There is probably a tendency to overprescribe all these classes of pharmacotherapeutic agents, especially the antianxiety drugs and the antidepressants. Normal fear responses and normal grief reactions do not require medication. Often these medications make such people feel even worse. A second trend, however, is seen as well. Once a given psychoactive agent is indicated, there is a tendency to *underdose* the patient. Doses should be gradually increased and given for a sufficient length of time so that the patient truly has been given an adequate trial before the drug is discontinued.

## Anticompulsive Disorder Agents

It is now clear that SRIs have a salubrious effect in some patients with an obsessive–compulsive disorder, perhaps especially with those who have a family history of this disorder.

**Interviews** are conducted for many purposes—research, education, selling merchandise, and moral persuasion, among others. Even when the interaction is intended to be therapeutic, such may not be the case. A good doctor–patient relationship sets the stage, but whether an interview or a series of interviews has a therapeutic outcome depends on many other factors. Outcome depends on the motivations of both parties, the capacities of both participants, the nature of the communication process, the experiences facilitated by the encounter, the resulting inner permission given by the patient to himself or herself to experiment with new patterns of action, the practice opportunities within the context of the interview to effect change, and the balance between resistance and assistance for change in the patient's environs. Psychotherapy is not limited to the process that occurs between a formally designated therapist and a patient. It occurs, for good or ill, during a patient's interaction with any physician.

## Psychotherapy Effects Change

Psychotherapy, if effective, facilitates change, a giving up or a modification of maladaptive responses and the acquisition of more adaptive behaviors. Without change at some level—biochemical, intrapsychic, behavioral, interpersonal—the patient stays sick. He or she holds to a dis-easing response pattern and maintains a character structure vulnerable to illness. Although therapists may use different theoretic frameworks for understanding human behavior, may belong to different schools of therapeutic intervention, and have different styles in their work, they are similar in their efforts to facilitate change.

## Process of Psychotherapy

### Awareness

The process of psychotherapy can be described. The therapeutic sequence discussed earlier (see Chap. 2) facilitates the process. As is the case with acquiring any new skill, whether walking or talking for a child, or farming or performing a surgical operation for an adult, the first step is increased **awareness**. Without awareness for the possibility of change, without awareness of possible options, without awareness of some of the determinants in these options, choices remain elusive. The effective therapist facilitates increased awareness, often in the face of resistance and unconscious if not conscious opposition from the patient. The evaluation process described earlier in this review not only sharpens diagnostic accuracy and enhances interviewing efficiency, but encourages increased awareness.

*Understanding*

From this awareness evolves **understanding**. It is not enough for the child to be aware of the possibility of walking. To walk, there must also be understanding of that process, whether acquired by imitation or formal study. As therapy proceeds, awareness fosters more complete understanding of the maladaptive process in question. Ultimately, more significant than the physician's understanding is the patient's understanding.

*Decision*

From this understanding, a range of possible alternatives comes into view, and after due consideration, **decision**. To continue our analogy, awareness of the possibility of walking, understanding the process of walking, does not make a walker. Insight in and of itself is not enough. To walk requires the decision to walk. To effect change requires a decision as to the what, the how, and the when of change.

*Practice*

Acquiring and integrating a new behavior requires **practice**. The effective therapist encourages and supports such practice, again often in the face of resistance. Any new behavior is unskilled, awkward, and does not feel natural. The new behavior also opposes, so to speak, the dynamics in the neurotic solution to the conflict. Beyond this, change when manifested may be resisted by the patient's surround. For example, a male patient with a dependent personality recovering from depression may experience resistance from his wife and children as he moves behaviorally toward independence.

*New Behavior*

Finally, with sufficient practice, the circle is complete. The **new behavior** now integrated feels natural. The new behavior allows a **new level of awareness**. Having learned to walk, no longer having to pay attention to the walking *per se*, the child becomes aware of a whole new world. Many patients avoid change because, to oversimplify, they wait for the feeling to change first. They say, for example, "When I no longer feel so terrified, then I'll be able to get on the elevator." Change in feeling comes after practice, not before. Others avoid change because they obsess, waiting for the "right" decision, the "perfect" solution, the "answer" that has no consequences other than the relief of symptoms.

## Comparison of Therapies

The emphasis may be different between therapies. Traditional psychoanalysis emphasizes awareness and understanding and tends to assume that the patient will work through the decision/practice part of the change cycle. With appropriately selected patients, this can occur. Certain behavior therapies tend to ignore awareness and understanding, focus on a particular decision often prescribed, and detail a schedule for practice. Again, with appropriate selection, there can be good outcome. Most psychoanalysts and behavior therapists would object to this somewhat stereotyped description, and appropriately so. Neither completely ignores the principles of the other. The principle of individual response specificity would suggest that some patients are more likely to benefit from one method than another. Controlled studies of therapeutic efficacy are beginning to demonstrate the validity of this statement.

# CHARACTERISTICS OF EFFECTIVE PHYSICIANS

The following represents a summary of the characteristics of effective physicians based on outcome studies—that is, given a group of physicians whose patients have an effective outcome by some measure, what are their characteristics compared with those physicians whose patients by the same measure do not have a comparable outcome? Interestingly, the results of these studies suggest comparable characteristics, whether the study relates to pediatricians and the rates of recurring otitis media in their patients, family physicians and maintenance of weight reduction by their patients, surgeons and morbidity rates after gallbladder surgery, psychiatrists and rate of rehospitalization of schizophrenic patients, therapists and measured improvement in their depressed patients with cognitive psychotherapy, and so forth.

It is interesting to notice what is not significantly different between the two groups of physicians in a given study. There do not seem to be significant differences in any cognitive measurement (e.g., IQ, grades in medical school, or performance on traditional national testing examinations). Apparently, the system that selects individuals into medicine and the system that educates them accomplishes the cognitive mission. Physicians learn what they need to know. In these studies, at least, there appears to be no significant differences between the two groups in this domain. However, there are differences in other dimensions.

## Provides Appropriate Nurturing

First, the effective physician is appropriately nurturing, that is, appropriately supportive. Some physicians tend to be "too nurturing," taking a stance that might be characterized in the following message to the patient: "I care about you. You simply should trust me and place yourself in my hands. Don't worry. I know what is in your best interest." Others tend to be "insufficiently nurturing." Their message may be characterized in this manner: "I know what to do. I intend to do it. You follow my instructions. If you don't get better, it's essentially your fault." Patronizing communication is characteristic of the first example, whereas blaming communication is characteristic of the second. Neither is appropriately nurturing in most instances.

## Provides Cognitive Model

Based on the data, the second characteristic of effective physicians is even more powerful in the statistical sense than the previous one. An effective physician is extraordinarily skilled in providing a cognitive model so that the patient understands the disease process. This is not surprising; the patient who understands hypertension is more likely to follow the antihypertensive regimen than one who does not, especially through periods when there may be no symptoms and even side effects from the medication. With psychotherapy, despite what adamant adherents to given schools of psychotherapy may proclaim, there are no data from any given theoretic model that show it to be consistently more powerful than another. A therapist who uses transactional analysis does not necessarily have better outcomes than one who uses the model of Freudian psychoanalysis, or another who uses a model from learning theory. The nihilist may jump to the conclusion that it is not necessary to have a model at all. But this is not the case either. Apparently, what these good therapists have in common is some model of understanding, a model they understand very well and are able to use, and especially a model they can communicate to their patients with consistency from interview to interview. What follows is that the patient achieves an understanding.

## Involves Patient in Problem Solving

Third, what seems to emerge from the evidence is that the effective physician is skilled in involving the patient in problem solving. This is in striking contrast to the "sick" role as defined by Western culture, which tends to exempt patients from being responsible for their illness and simply expects them to comply with the recommendations of the health expert. It is also in striking contrast to the all-too-frequently observed process of the physician making his or her diagnosis after evaluation and simply prescribing a therapeutic regimen. Involving certain patients in the problem-solving process requires considerable skill.

## Makes Accurate Diagnoses

Finally, effective physicians make accurate diagnoses. Note the plural: they rediagnose the patient with every visit. They place at axis I the disease bringing the patient to the encounter. Their diagnoses are multidimensional. For example, "Here is a generalized anxiety disorder with a superimposed adjustment reaction and anxious mood in a patient with compulsive and avoidant characteristics and well managed essential hypertension who recently had a friend killed in the Oklahoma bombing." One month later the patient returns. "Today, I see exudative tonsillitis probably secondary to strep in a patient with compulsive and avoidant characteristics with well managed essential hypertension, a generalized anxiety disorder, recovering from the adjustment reaction with anxious mood in response to the death of a friend. In the center of the biopsychosocial model stands my patient and her diseases. My evaluation and my management plan will proceed from within that framework."

The modality that creates the characteristics of the more competent physician, in considerable measure, clearly is **effective communication**.

# INTERPERSONAL OUTCOME

## Self-Esteem

A positive outcome between two people can be seen as depending on four factors. The first relates to the degree of **self-esteem** brought to the encounter by both parties. Self-esteem is highlighted here as an attribute of a normal, nonneurotic, emotionally healthy person, that is, a genital character. Emotionally healthy people are simply more likely to have a positive outcome. This is true whether the issue is communication between a father and a son, a mother and a daughter, a husband and a wife, two colleagues, or a physician and a patient. Although a physician cannot be responsible for the degree of self-esteem brought to the interaction by the patient, the physician is responsible for the self-esteem that he or she brings to the practice of medicine. This dimension is not the focus of this section, nor can it be. Still, it is no accident that studies show repeatedly that genital characters tend to have better outcome in their encounters. Yet, even if both parties bring considerable self-esteem, that does not necessarily predict a favorable outcome in itself.

## Communication Skills

The second factor is **communication**—to what degree both parties possess and use specific communication skills. This is the major theme of this section.

# Rules of the Encounter

The third factor is what **rules** the two people bring to the encounter. What is the nature of these rules, and to what degree have they been contracted explicitly? Certain rules are inherent in some of the concepts previously discussed. Patients declare their dis-ease, not the physician. The physician's task is to decide with the patient in what way the patient is dis-eased and by what strategy the dis-ease might be alleviated. Contracting is a kind of rule making. A review of those pertinent paragraphs in the discussion of the therapeutic sequence might be in order (see Chap. 2).

Other rules are more subtle. To exemplify, I would ask the reader the following question, "When growing up, what were the rules in your house regarding doors?" All families have such rules. What were the rules regarding bathroom doors or bedroom doors? Was the rule, for example, that the adults in the family could go through any door at any time, but children could not? It should be noted that there is not necessarily a right rule, but any rule has its own set of consequences.

Shifting context, I might ask, "What are the rules in your office regarding doors?" The physician who closes the door announces, "I am in charge of the door." Several studies demonstrate that physicians who shut their door obtain more accurate and more confidential information during evaluation than physicians who allow office personnel to close the door. That office personnel close the door also means that they can open it; the behavior says, "Patient, you can expect an interruption at any time, and whatever you are saying may be overheard."

# Support

Finally, the fourth factor predicting interpersonal outcome relates to the **support from the surround**. This is a whole topic unto itself. It includes how the phone is answered, how appointments are scheduled, what information is obtained at the time of appointment by the receptionist, how that information is communicated, and how the office is arranged. Of increasing concern is whether managed care supports or does not support the physician–patient relationship. Does the gate keeper? Does the insurance policy? Does the billing office? Let us return to communication.

To quote a famous and for many a sacred book, "In the beginning was the Word." However that may be interpreted, we must say that human interaction usually does not begin with the word. It begins with the face. It continues with the feeling. The word comes later. This is true for the developing infant; it is true for the conversation around the breakfast table. It is also true for the physician–patient interaction. This fact shapes the therapeutic sequence. But when words come, there is indeed considerable impact.

# COMMUNICATION

Physician communication can be classified moment by moment with high reliability by judges into one of the following communication modes. The semantics in the sentence and the accompanying nonverbal behavior determine the category.

## Types of Communicators

### Placating Communication

**Placators** are prepared to agree with whatever the other says. They seem to say, "What counts here is what you think or believe or feel, not what I think or believe or feel." Placators have difficulty with confrontation, sometimes even when this takes the form of a clarifying question.

### Patronizing Communication

The **patronizer** seems to operate from the posture, "I know what is best for you, and I will decide what is in your best interest." If placators diminish themselves, patronizers diminish the other. This communication is often difficult to counter because it seems to come with the metamessage, "I really care about you, and being older or wiser or the expert in this situation, you should depend on me."

### Blaming Communication

**Blamers** seem to take the stance, "Whatever is wrong here, it is obviously your fault." Blamers invite guilt. "If you would only correct what you are doing wrong or do what I tell you to do, everything would be better."

### Rationalizing Communication

**Rationalizers** give detailed reasons, often after the fact. They take an action or make a statement and then justify that action or statement. Conversely, some give the explanation or build the argument before the behavior.

### Distracting Communication

**Distracters** do not seem to keep track of the topic at hand. Their own associations simply intrude into what the other hopes will be a goal-directed conversation. In some instances, distraction is a deliberate method to take the conversation in a different direction.

*Leveling Communication*

Leveling communication has three characteristics. The first is that of **ownership**. The semantics of the sentence make it clear that the speaker owns the belief, the feeling, the thought. The speaker acknowledges that what the speaker hears from the other is what the speaker hears, and not what the other said. This is typically conveyed by accurate use of pronouns.

The second is **clarity**. Clarity is particularly evident in the use of verbs. The speaker does not confuse believing with thinking, feeling, seeing, hearing, knowing, or acting.

The third characteristic is a method that conveys that the **message sent is the message received**. The only way I can know whether the other has heard what I have said is to hear what I have said back. My patient cannot know that I have heard what they have said unless I have said it back. Conversely, I cannot know whether the patient has heard what I have said unless I hear it back from them. Nodding one's head or a short phrase of agreement is simply not sufficient, especially when communication is of considerable significance and import. Again, communication between physicians and their patients is usually of considerable import.

In studies of physician–patient communication, physicians who are more effective are skilled in using *all* of the above modes as appropriate to a given situation. **Leveling**, however, is the **characteristic and predominant mode**. Still, there are times to placate. The gratuitous "we" of patronizing communication can be reassuring. There are situations in which the other modes are useful as well. Unfortunately, studies have shown that the most frequent communication used by physicians is blaming. Judges frequently rate blaming communication based on the nonverbal accompaniments to the sentence. Physicians are often unaware of their blaming demeanor. The second most common is patronizing; the third most common is rationalizing, and the fourth is leveling. In general, physicians as a group are not particularly skillful communicators.

## Listening in Communication

**Transformational grammatics** postulates that for every event in the world there is a structure in the deep language system such that a native user of that language can utter a sentence that has the quality of synonymy, that is, it is unambiguous and does not leave significant questions in the mind of the listener. For example, the statement, "That man over there is hitting that table with the flat of his right hand" is considerably less ambiguous than, "Somebody is hitting something." The skillful listener notices the ambiguities in the transformations. Particularly when communication is of import, usually the case in the physician–patient interaction, inquiries are made in such a way as to clarify the ambiguity.

Hence, the physician learns to listen for **deletions**. A patient says, "I have this pain in my belly." The deletions include, *When* does the patient have the pain? *Where* exactly is it? *What* triggers the pain? *How* long does the pain last? *What* is the nature of the pain? So far, all this may seem obvious, but deletions can be much harder to identify. There are deletions connected to adjectives and to adverbs. Another patient states, "My husband says I am the worst nag in the world." It is not clear to whom he says it. It is not clear to whom she is being compared in being the worst nag. It is not even clear what "world" is being talked about. If the listener is not careful, he or she will fill in the deletion. It would be easy to assume that the husband is talking to the wife, your patient, but that may not be the case.

The skillful listener also listens for **generalizations**. "Somebody" and "something" in the sentence above are generalizations. Another patient says, "My husband always interrupts me." Another reports, "I'm nervous all the time." "Always" and "all" are generalizations. With a generalization, specificity cannot be discerned, and it is therefore difficult to arrive at a specific plan for intervention.

Finally, a skillful listener hears **distortions**. Within the framework of transformational grammatics, the most common distortion is a nominalization—turning a process into a thing, or, put differently, turning a verb into a noun. A thing can be put into a wheelbarrow. There is no such thing as "a marriage." A marriage is a process. A process turned into an event tends to become immutable, unchangeable. A medical student says to her physician, "I made a terrible decision when I came to medical school." A skillful physician might say, "What keeps you from undeciding?," turning decision, a thing, back into a process. Change is possible!

Physicians should remember that most of our "diseases" are not "things," either. Diabetes is a process, not a thing. Schizophrenia is a process, not a thing. Coronary artery disease is a process, not a thing. A physician who says, "By working together, I think we can bring your diabetes into better control" is uttering a different statement with significantly different meaning than one who says, "Your diabetes is out of control." Which physician, would you think, has better compliance?

An efficient physician listens carefully, notes the regulator indicating the patient is through talking, and often uses a word or a short phrase to clarify the ambiguity. A patient states, "I want to stop taking this medicine." The physician responds, "Because?" Another patient says, "I've had this pain for a long time." The physician responds, "Days? Weeks? Months?" A word or a phrase also fills a smaller space in talk time. Evaluation, obviously, involves data gathering, and most of the data are in the patient. Therefore, it should not be surprising that studies show that the greater percentage of the time that physicians talk, the less data they gather given the same block of time.

## Talking in Communication

Physicians tend to underestimate considerably the percentage of time they spend talking during the physician–patient encounter. In one study, physician talk time was 70% and that for patients was 30%, but the same physicians, on average, estimated that they talked 20% of the time while their patients talked 80% of the time. Interestingly, their patients were more accurate in their judgments. They estimated that they themselves talked 20% of the time and their doctors talked 80% of the time.

In the same study, the physician–patient interaction was interrupted 30% of the time either by someone coming through the door or the telephone. Furthermore, the patient's response to the physician's opening question was interrupted 77% of the time, and within 15 seconds 63% of the time. In general, female physicians talk less during their physician–patient encounters compared with male physicians. Therefore, they tend to get more complete and more accurate histories.

The physician's task is to help the patient talk in complete sentences. When the sentence is complete without deletions, generalizations, or distortions, what usually follows is understanding. With understanding comes at least the possibility for intervention, for change. In this sense all physicians working with patients must be psychotherapists.

Medical students bring their communication styles to medical school. They typically copy the professional communication styles they hear from their mentors, regardless of whether they are effective. So, learning here, almost without exception, means unlearning first. To become an effective communicator means listening to oneself, preferably through the technology of videotape and often with someone skilled in its use. This is an important task for physicians, because effective communication is the base on which the physician–patient relationship is structured. It is the base on which all therapies are built.

# TYPES OF PSYCHOTHERAPY

Before reviewing the various types of psychotherapy, it should be noted that in the last decade studies of therapeutic outcome are demonstrating the significant effect of appropriately conducted psychotherapy. The studies involve control groups, counterbalanced design, reliable measurements, and careful statistical analysis—the usual requirements in scientific medicine. Of course, clinical experience has for years suggested such an effect. This kind of research is just beginning. Much remains to be done. The results of such studies seem to show a greater effect than therapeutic nihilists might have anticipated, but less effect than therapeutic enthusiasts would have predicted.

## Hypnotherapy

Historically, hypnosis was one of the earliest psychotherapies. It was used initially to effect suggestion during the hypnotic state or to accomplish psychological catharsis and abreaction. The technique also can facilitate dynamic understanding of the pathologic process. In the modern era, it is probably used most successfully for control of pain and for early intervention with conversion or dissociative disorders. The technique tends to foster dependent attitudes in certain patients. For others it savors of magic, and to others it seems to threaten their need for control. Of course, all effective therapies have potential adverse side effects.

## Relaxation Therapy and Biofeedback

The teaching of relaxation techniques also has a long history. A more sophisticated version uses biofeedback techniques, although the effect of biofeedback is probably not related simply to skeletal muscle relaxation in all instances. There are reports of therapeutic effect in many kinds of patients, but most consistently in patients with generalized anxiety accompanied by generalized muscular tension and in patients with specific psychophysiology syndromes, in particular, tension headache, and certain varieties of hypertension.

## Individual Psychotherapies

**Psychoanalysis** or psychoanalytic-oriented therapy makes considerable use of the technique of **free association**, which encourages patients to put into words whatever comes to their minds without censuring. At first, this is difficult for most patients to do; however, over time, this technique carries the possibility of fostering more complete understanding of the pathologic process.

Related to psychoanalysis is a variety of **dynamic psychotherapies**. Here also, there is considerable emphasis on increasing awareness and developing understanding. As is the case with psychoanalysis, transference may be fostered and used through interpretation to bring greater understanding to the pathologic process. Transference refers to the unconscious tendency of the patient to respond to the therapist as if he or she were someone else, a significant other in the patient's present or past.

The concept of fixation is also characteristic of many of these therapies, namely, that maladaptive behavior patterns are old patterns that persist from specific points in time of psychological development and revolve around certain issue. Returning to those situations and events in the patient's past history, reexamining them, reinterpreting them, and identifying their role in the present is a process effecting change.

**Supportive psychotherapy** emphasizes the development of a more effective support system for the patient in his family setting or work setting. It also seeks to discover the more healthy behaviors in the patient and encourages their elaboration. Uncovering the past, making the unconscious conscious, is not emphasized, and may even be avoided. There is, of course, a supportive element to all effective therapies.

**Educational psychotherapy** is a term given to that intervention that focuses primarily on educational techniques. There is also an element of education in all therapies.

**Behavior therapy** using the principles of learning theory also has many variations, but focuses specifically in some fashion on a program of practice of behaviors to help the patient extinguish old, inadequate responses or learn new, more adaptive ones. Some forms of behavior therapy may be particularly helpful to patients who have phobias or in patients who clearly need to alter specific destructive habit patterns (e.g., overeating, smoking).

## Group Psychotherapy

The group psychotherapies are as varied as the individual therapies. They share in common patients working together in the context of a group. Certain therapists use a psychoanalytic theoretic background with an emphasis on developing an understanding of each member of the group or an understanding of the group process as a whole. Others may be more active and experiential, for example, those who use psychodrama. Conjoint marital therapy, that is, working with both husband and wife, might be viewed as the smallest group therapy possible. Family therapy focuses on therapy with the whole family. Particular indications for these techniques may be in those situations in which pathologic interactions occurring between the dyad or between members of the family perpetuate pathologic processes. Group psychotherapy has an advantage in that it provides the patient with a particular opportunity to practice such new behaviors as more openly sharing feelings, responding to angry confrontations, and so forth, in a safe and supportive setting and with people who are not part of the patient's family or work group.

## Self-Help Groups

These groups can be extraordinarily helpful in some situations in fostering therapeutic outcome. Perhaps the best known is Alcoholics Anonymous. It is effective in helping a significant percentage of alcoholics maintain abstinence. Other groups have been modeled after Alcoholics Anonymous, including such groups as

Narcotics Anonymous and Weight Watchers. There are self-help groups made up of people who have recovered from severe mental illness, groups that share in common a particular kind of chronic disease or having undergone similar surgery (e.g., colostomy, mastectomy), or share in common the death of a child or the loss of a marital partner.

Finally, given the primary intent of this review, it might be useful in closing to say that self-help groups have been formed by people who share in common the anticipated taking of national certifying or competency examinations, and physicians who share in common a motive to improve their competence, increase the efficiency and effectiveness of their group practice, enhance the health status of their patients, and move their intervention toward cost containment.

# Appendix

These comments refer to the set of photographs on page 19. First read the text; next read the faces. Finally, review these comments. (The numbered paragraphs refer to the corresponding numbered photographs.)

1. Universal face of **acceptance/comfort**. Face looks expressionless. Facial muscles are relaxed, especially the muscles about the mouth. Mouth is often slightly open. (Example: The physician has just said, "I would like to do a physical examination, now." Patient replies, "Fine." The patient's word and the patient's face, that is, the subjective evidence and the objective evidence, are congruent. There is no need for further follow-up.) When accompanied by a tense, thin lip or tensing of the masseter muscle, acceptance is being simulated. The face says, in essence, "I'm hiding from you, and perhaps from myself, what I am really feeling or thinking."

2. Universal face of **disgust**. Note the down-turned corners of the mouth and the increased prominence of the nasolabial folds. With extreme disgust, the nose may wrinkle and the nares flare. Disgust is an emotion registered in the lower half of the face. (Example: The physician has just said, "I would like to do a physical examination now." Patient replies, "Fine." In contrast to number 1, the subjective and objective evidence are incongruent. Physician might follow with, "There is something about the physical that is bothersome?") Disgust is often presented relatively briefly, in flashes. It indicates disgust with the event at hand, whether listening to or observing another, talking, or thinking. The face says "I would like to be rid of this."

3. Universal face of moderate **surprise**. Note the wrinkled forehead, the somewhat raised eyebrows and the somewhat open mouth. (Example; The physician has just said, "Your blood pressure is normal." The patient says, "Really." The physician's response might be, "You seem surprised.") Surprise is often flashed relatively briefly. Skilled communicators look for surprise in the listener and typically interrupt their flow of communication by inquiring about the surprise. Key information is often uncovered in this fashion that otherwise would be missed. The upper half of the face of surprise is used in our culture as

an emblem indicating, "I'm asking you a question." When combined with disgust, it is an emblem of skepticism. (Example: A physician has just said, "Your blood pressure is normal," or "I think we can discontinue your medication." To the facial emblematic reply, the physician might say, "To me you look a bit skeptical." Again, critical information may be uncovered. Often compliance is increased by dealing with the underlying doubt. Note the leveling communication; the physician did not say, "Why are you skeptical?") Disgust combined with a smile in our culture is often emblematic of disdain or scorn.

4. The universal face of **joy**. Note that both the eyes and the mouth are smiling. Joy involves the whole face. (Example: The physician has just said, "Your blood pressure is normal." The patient has responded, "Good." The physician then might say, "I think you're happy to hear that.") When the lower half of the face of joy is presented, namely, a smiling mouth in the context of initially meeting someone, it is an emblem meaning, "I intend to be friendly." It does not mean, "I am happy." A smiling mouth is a common simulator. When accompanied by the upper half of the facies in Photographs 5, 6, or 7, it presents a confusing, incongruent facial behavior. The smiling mouth tends to deceive the observer. In a sense, it hides what the eyes are saying. When well practiced, the patients themselves may be unaware of the underlying distressing emotion signaled by the eyes.

5. The universal face of profound **fear/anxiety**. In clinical practice, less intense facial expression of fear/anxiety is much more common than this particular example. When congruent, patients tend to use the word "fear" when they recognize the stress that is triggering the fear. When patients speak about feeling "anxious," commonly they do not connect feeling anxious with the idea of feeling scared, or they cannot identify the source of their anxiety, or both. Contrast this face to the face of surprise, with which there is some similarity. In addition to the transverse wrinkles across the forehead, note the furrowing between the eyes. This is produced by the corrugator muscle, sometimes called the muscle of distress. Also note that white appears above the iris. In many patients, the lower lid is also tense, producing an effect not previously noted. With anxiety, the mouth is not only open, but often the teeth are seen, either the lower, the upper, or both. The lower half of the face of disgust and the upper half of the face of anxiety constitutes a blend. The face suggests, "I'm disgusted with my anxiety."

6. The universal face of **anger**. The head juts forward, the eyes narrow and are focused; the corrugator furrows the brow and the teeth are bared. Display rules teach that this degree of undisguised anger should be minimized. Therefore, the mouth often is closed although still tense, and the head does not jut forward but is held in position, tensely and rigidly. When the lower half of the face is relaxed but the upper half of the face appears angry, it is emblematic of thinking. Anger plus disgust

often appear as a blend. This blend is particularly distressing to a child. It says, "I'm not only angry with you, I'm disgusted with you as well, and I might as well be rid of you!" If the mouth is smiling but the eyes indicate anger, the smile is a simulator hiding the anger.

7. The universal face of **sadness**. This is the only primary emotion that does not maintain eye contact. The muscles of the face become somewhat flaccid, the head drops, the eyelids drop, and the patient looks down. With intense sadness and before the appearance of tears, the corrugator is again brought into play. (Example: The physician has just said, "How is your marriage?" The patient does not respond verbally, shakes his head slightly, and appears as in the picture. Depending on the nature of the relationship, the physician might say, "To me you look like you are about to cry.") The face of clinical depression, in contrast to the face of sadness and grief, includes elements of fear or anger as a blend.

These are the seven primary emotions. Expressors are universal when presented in an undisguised fashion. There are many blends, and there are facial sequences. It should be noted that there is no universal face of shame or guilt. This is also true of secondary emotions. Emblems, simulators, and adaptors are not universal either, but tend to be consistent in meaning in a given individual.

8. A common **emblem of thinking**. Note the upper half of the face of anger, together with a relaxed mouth and the position of the finger. (Example: The physician has just asked, "How would you describe this pain?" The patient is thinking. The physician is well advised to remain silent, not repeat the question, not elaborate, but give this patient time to respond.)

9. A face of anxiety plus a self-nurturing or self-reassuring gesture. This hand gesture is an **adaptor**. In this patient, the adaptor says, "I attempt to handle my anxiety by reassuring myself. If you are an observant and understanding physician, that's what I'm going to need from you." In our society, the reassuring, self-grooming gesture of men is different from comparable gestures in women.

10. A **respiratory avoidance response** plus a hint of sadness. The response may include sniffing or clearing the throat. Note the stroking gesture of the forefinger across the nares. This comes close to being a universal emblem, and indicates, "I am in some measure uncomfortable and wish to be rid of this." The gesture may be in response to what the physician has just said or what the patient has just said, is about to say, or is thinking. (It also might mean that the patient has a cold!) Sometimes, it suggests the opposite of what the patient has just said. (Example: This patient has headaches, which he labels muscular tension headaches. He believes they are related to stress. In attempting to identify the stress, the physician already has asked about his work and his marriage. The patient's verbal and nonverbal responses did not suggest stress in these areas. The physician then

asked about his children. This patient first described his youngest, a daughter. His face looked very much like Photograph 4. [Ordinarily, patients start with their eldest.] Then, he talked matter-of-factly about his next oldest. Finally he says, "Then of course, there is my eldest, he's 21 and in college and he's doing OK." But, while saying that, he appears as in this picture. Given the sequence, one stress area for this patient is almost certainly connected with his eldest son. The patient may or may not recognize this initially.)

Again, there are many blends. There are many sequences of nonverbal behavior involving face, hands, feet, and body posture. These sequences can be considered as sentences. As stated in the text, the skillful communicator overcomes his or her recognition rules, trains himself or herself to read such sentences, and correlates these behaviors with the subtleties of verbal language. Also, the skillful communicator becomes familiar with his or her own characteristic emblems, regulators, adapters, and simulators and knows his or her propensities for congruence or incongruence with each of the primary emotions.

# PSYCHIATRY AND BEHAVIORAL MEDICINE QUESTIONS

DIRECTIONS: Each set of numbered items or incomplete statements in this section is followed by answers or by completions of the statement. Select the ONE lettered answer or completion that is BEST in each case.

1. This review is organized around the

   (A) disciplinary assumption
   (B) biopsychosocial concept of disease
   (C) subject assumption
   (D) biopsychosocial model of disease
   (E) tasks of the health professional assumption

2. The attitudinal task speaks of a *psychological need profile*. Physicians tend to organize their practice of medicine to gratify this profile. They expend time and energy to achieve one need in contrast to another. In my judgment, I would score the highest on which of the following?

   (A) Need for power, influence, and control: the political scale
   (B) Need for economic return: the economic scale
   (C) Need to know in order to understand: the scientific scale
   (D) Need to relate to people: the social scale
   (E) Need to experience pleasurable feeling: the aesthetic scale

3. My feeling response to Question 2 is

   (A) acceptance
   (B) anger
   (C) anxiety
   (D) disgust
   (E) sadness

**4.** The biopsychosocial model suggests that the expected emotional and behavioral response to the category of stress termed "the unexpected" would be

**(A)** anxiety/fear and avoidant or fleeing behavior
**(B)** anxiety/fear and compulsive or assertive behavior
**(C)** anxiety/fear and orienting behavior
**(D)** surprise and orienting behavior
**(E)** surprise and avoidant or fleeing behavior

**5.** Which of the following statements concerning mental illness is most accurate?

**(A)** About one in four people during a lifetime will be hospitalized in a psychiatric hospital for mental illness
**(B)** Rates of admissions and discharges of patients to and from state mental hospitals are decreasing
**(C)** The most common diagnosis for patients with mental illness seen in ambulatory care medical settings is alcoholism
**(D)** The number of patients resident in county and state mental hospitals over the past decade has increased
**(E)** Approximately 25% to 30% of all visits to ambulatory care settings in the United States are related directly to mental illness

**6.** A surgical resident making early morning rounds of patients scheduled for elective surgery during the day makes one of the following opening statements to each patient as he enters. Which statement most clearly suggests the concept of stimulus–response specificity?

**(A)** "Good morning. How was your night?"
**(B)** "I know that you are a little anxious about the surgery. Would you like to talk about it?"
**(C)** "Well, how are you feeling this morning?"
**(D)** "Anything you would like to talk about this morning?"
**(E)** "Well, we're all set for your surgery. Are you?"

**7.** Which statement most clearly suggests the concept of individual–response specificity?

**(A)** "Anything you would like to talk about this morning?"
**(B)** "Good morning. How was your night?"
**(C)** "I know you are a little anxious about the surgery. Would you like to talk about it?"
**(D)** "Well, how are you feeling this morning?"
**(E)** "Well, we're all set for your surgery. Are you?"

8. The leading actual cause of death in the United States is related to which of the following?

    (A) Alcohol and illicit drugs
    (B) Diet and activity
    (C) Firearms
    (D) Microbes
    (E) Tobacco

9. During the first moments of an initial visit to a family physician, a 24-year-old man licks his lips and with a tremulous voice states, "Well, Doctor, it's good to meet you. I suppose that you are interested in why I'm here?" The physician nods and the patient continues, "Well, there is no problem really. I'm just here for a regular checkup." Which of the following statements is the best response that the physician should give?

    (A) "You are obviously anxious. What's bothering you?"
    (B) "Is there anything in particular that you'd like me to check?"
    (C) "Any particular reason that you decided to have a checkup right now?"
    (D) "I'm wondering if you're feeling a little uneasy."
    (E) "So there is nothing in particular and you're just here for a regular checkup. Right?"

10. An experienced pediatrician has completed his initial evaluation of a 9-year-old boy brought to the office by the boy's mother. The pediatrician has interviewed the mother. Given the evidence from the history and the physician, the pediatrician suspects that the boy has attention deficit disorder with hyperactivity. Other possibilities include hyperthyroidism and petit mal epilepsy. Which of the following is most likely to be helpful to the pediatrician in the diagnosis and management of this patient?

    (A) A blood chemistry battery of tests
    (B) Consultation with the patient's teacher, who can describe the patient's behavior
    (C) Electroencephalographic examination
    (D) Referral to a clinical psychologist for psychological tests
    (E) Referral to a neurologist for a detailed neurologic examination

**11.** While reviewing an electroencephalographic tracing from an adult patient with a long history of convulsive disorder, a physician notes considerable delta activity. The patient most likely

(A) fell asleep during the tracing
(B) has diffuse brain damage
(C) has the petit mal variety of epilepsy
(D) is entering a toxic delirium
(E) may have a space-occupying lesion

**12.** Which of the following accounts for the fewest number of cases of mental retardation in the United States?

(A) Down's syndrome
(B) Perinatal infections and early childhood encephalitides
(C) Phenylketonuria, Gaucher's disease, cretinism, Hurler's syndrome, and kernicterus
(D) Prematurity and birth trauma
(E) Primary mental retardation

**13.** Which of the following statements best characterizes patients with anorexia nervosa?

(A) They commonly report symptoms of hypersomnolence and lethargy
(B) They complain bitterly of nausea
(C) They frequently report feeling fat when objectively emaciated
(D) They are more commonly adolescent boys than adolescent girls
(E) They rarely die from this disorder

**14.** Of the following childhood disorders, psychogenesis is clearly most prominent in

(A) conduct disorder, aggressive socialized type
(B) attention deficit–hyperactivity disorder
(C) infantile autism
(D) sleep terrors
(E) Tourette's disorder

**15.** A house officer in the psychiatry department sees a 30-year-old man in the emergency department. The man has been hospitalized previously for a schizophrenic disorder, paranoid type. On this particular occasion, the man presents with all of the symptoms listed below. Which of these symptoms is most suggestive of a delirium (acute brain syndrome)?

   (A) Clouding of consciousness and disorientation
   (B) Concrete thinking
   (C) Persecutory delusions
   (D) Speech bordering on incoherence
   (E) Visual hallucinations

**16.** In contrast to alcohol withdrawal syndrome with delirium, alcohol hallucinosis is characterized by

   (A) a disturbed sleep–wake cycle
   (B) autistic thinking
   (C) clouding of consciousness
   (D) comparative absence of physiologic withdrawal symptoms
   (E) visual hallucinations

**17.** For people older than 65 years of age, the most common form of dementia is

   (A) Alzheimer's disease
   (B) arteriosclerotic dementia
   (C) multiple-infarct dementia
   (D) normal-pressure hydrocephalus
   (E) uremic encephalopathy

**18.** All of the following substances produce a withdrawal syndrome EXCEPT

   (A) barbiturates
   (B) caffeine
   (C) cocaine
   (D) opioids
   (E) tobacco

**19.** The intoxication most likely confused with an acute schizophrenic disorder is that produced by

(A) alcohol
(B) amphetamines
(C) barbiturates
(D) cocaine
(E) lysergic acid diethylamide

**20.** The possibility of suicide must be considered in all of the following conditions. In which condition is it LEAST likely?

(A) Alcoholism
(B) Bipolar disorder, mixed type
(C) Delirium (acute brain syndrome)
(D) Dementia with a depression
(E) Schizophreniform disorder

**21.** Which of the following statements regarding schizophrenic disorders is most accurate?

(A) An example of a primary symptom, according to Bleuler, is a persecutory delusion
(B) Process schizophrenia has a better prognosis than reactive schizophrenia
(C) Hebephrenia is more common than catatonia
(D) Schizophrenia affects 1% to 3% of the population
(E) Schizophrenia with a chronic course shows deterioration toward dementia

**22.** A genetic component probably plays a role in the genesis of all of the following mental disorders. However, the evidence is LEAST compelling in which of the following illnesses?

(A) Alzheimer's disease
(B) Huntington's chorea
(C) Manic–depressive disorder
(D) Panic disorder
(E) Schizophrenia

**23.** When compared with unipolar disorders, bipolar disorders

   **(A)** are less likely to respond to lithium during the acute phase
   **(B)** are less likely to benefit prophylactically from lithium treatment
   **(C)** are more common in women than in men
   **(D)** may have an acute episode precipitated by use of imipramine
   **(E)** occur in patients who are older

**24.** In primary care ambulatory settings, patients frequently have "depression" as their presenting complaint. In such instances, the most common diagnosis is

   **(A)** adjustment disorder with depressed mood
   **(B)** dysthymic disorder (depressive neurosis)
   **(C)** major depression with melancholia
   **(D)** manic–depressive illness (bipolar disorder)
   **(E)** uncomplicated grief in response to loss

**25.** Imipramine is the most likely drug of choice indicated in patients with

   **(A)** generalized anxiety disorders
   **(B)** panic disorder
   **(C)** obsessive–compulsive disorders
   **(D)** posttraumatic stress disorders
   **(E)** social phobias

**26.** A male patient diagnosed with a major depression with psychotic features is hospitalized. He is given a trial dose of imipramine (Tofranil), but is unresponsive. A decision is made to attempt to administer a different drug. In this situation, which one of the following would most likely be the drug of choice?

   **(A)** Amitriptyline (Elavil)
   **(B)** Desipramine (Norpramin)
   **(C)** Lithium carbonate (Eskalith)
   **(D)** Nortriptyline (Aventyl)
   **(E)** Phenelzine sulfate (Nardil)

**27.** A 32-year-old man reports difficulty maintaining an erection during intercourse with his wife. This situation has developed gradually over the past 3 years since his marriage at age 29. He had experienced no such difficulty before marriage. He reports noting full morning erections on wakening. He has had a sexual experience on a recent business trip and noted no difficulty with erection on that occasion. He says he is embarrassed about having this difficulty, and he frequently looks embarrassed as he gives his history to the physician. He volunteers no other symptoms of significance. Given the above information, the most appropriate tentative diagnosis would be

(A) adjustment disorder with anxious mood
(B) adjustment disorder with depressed mood
(C) latent ego-dystonic homosexuality
(D) male orgasmic disorder
(E) sexual arousal disorder

**28.** In which one of the following skin disorders are psychological factors of LEAST significance?

(A) Acne
(B) Dermatitis factitia
(C) Hyperhidrosis
(D) Rosacea
(E) Urticaria

**29.** Psychological factors are most significant etiologically in which one of the following skin disorders?

(A) Dermatitis factitia
(B) Hyperhidrosis
(C) Pemphigus
(D) Rosacea
(E) Urticaria

**30.** All of the following statements about electroconvulsive therapy are correct EXCEPT

(A) risk of mortality in patients with depression is considerably less than the risk of mortality in such patients who are untreated

(B) the most common complication is inducing a transient organic brain disorder

(C) the most commonly accepted indication for use is major depression

(D) it is contraindicated in patients with aortic aneurysms or coronary artery disease

(E) the use of muscle relaxants has decreased the incidence of compression fractures of the spine

**31.** Based on patient outcome studies, therapists with good outcome compared with therapists with poorer outcome are more likely to demonstrate

(A) higher scores on the psychiatry and neurology Board examinations

(B) a tendency to use patronizing communication

(C) a tendency to use psychopharmacologic agents less frequently

(D) skill in involving the patient in the problem-solving process

(E) use of the psychoanalytic model of therapy compared with the transactional analysis model of therapy

**32.** Which of the following statements about transference is correct?

(A) The unconscious tendency of the patient to respond to a situation in the present as if in some measure it were a situation from the past

(B) The unconscious tendency of the patient to respond to the physician as if he or she were someone else

(C) The unconscious tendency of the physician to respond to the patient as if he or she were someone else

(D) The conscious tendency of the patient to displace feelings felt toward others to the physician

(E) The conscious tendency of the physician to displace feelings felt toward others to the patient

33. Assume that the display rules taught by a culture also predict its recognition rules. Given that assumption, when comparing male physicians to female physicians, which of the following statements is most likely to be correct?

    (A) Male physicians are more likely to recognize anger in older women than in older men
    (B) Male physicians are more likely accurately to recognize anxiety in older men
    (C) Female physicians are more likely to recognize sadness than anger in older men
    (D) Female physicians are more likely to recognize anger in older women than in older men
    (E) Female physicians are more likely to recognize sadness in older men

34. A patient enters the dentist's office and says matter-of-factly, "I think I need to have a tooth pulled." Which of the following responses by the dentist most clearly suggests an evolving, associative interview? The dentist

    (A) nods, raises his eyebrows, and waits.
    (B) says, "Yes, you need a tooth pulled."
    (C) says, "The tooth must be bothering you."
    (D) nods, gestures toward the examining chair, and after the patient is seated, says, "Well, let's have a look."
    (E) says, "Where does it hurt?"

35. Careful evaluation of a man who complains of feeling discouraged about his marriage indicates that the problem mainly seems to relate to pathologic communication patterns between the husband and wife. This suggests referral for evaluation of which of the following?

    (A) Conjoint marital therapy
    (B) Educational psychotherapy for the couple
    (C) Group therapy for the couple
    (D) Group therapy for the patient
    (E) Psychoanalytically oriented psychotherapy for the patient

*Questions 36–38*

A resident in Internal Medicine enters an emergency department to see a patient, a man approximately 43 years of age, who is sitting on the examining table. The man's shoulders are slumped, his head and eyes are cast downward, and his eyes are red. He looks up slowly and after a deep sigh says, "I'm sorry to bother you, Doctor, but I have to talk to someone. I've been so discouraged and depressed lately that I'm afraid I might try to kill myself."

**36.** At this point, the patient is exhibiting

   **(A)** verbal and behavioral evidence for anxiety
   **(B)** verbal and behavioral evidence for sadness
   **(C)** verbal and behavioral evidence for anger
   **(D)** only behavioral evidence for anxiety
   **(E)** only behavioral evidence for sadness

**37.** Given the above information, what is the most effective immediate response the physician should give?

   **(A)** "Don't worry, you're not bothering me."
   **(B)** "Have you ever tried to kill yourself?"
   **(C)** "What is it exactly that you are afraid might happen?"
   **(D)** "You look and feel depressed. Do you have any idea why you are so discouraged?"
   **(E)** "Would you like to talk to a psychiatrist?"

**38.** Given the available evidence concerning this patient, which of the following is the most likely diagnosis?

   **(A)** Dysthymic disorder
   **(B)** Major depressive disorder
   **(C)** Mood disorder due to a general medical condition
   **(D)** Schizoaffective disorder
   **(E)** Uncomplicated bereavement

*Questions 39–41*

A well-dressed woman in her early thirties consults a pediatrician for the first time. While fidgeting with her hands, she states, "I want to talk to you about my 7-year-old daughter. I'm worried about her. She hasn't done anything like this since she was 2 or 3 years old. Last week, she wet the bed on two nights. I've been reading, and frankly I'm afraid of what this might mean." The woman pauses and looks at the pediatrician with wide-open eyes.

39. Noting the behavioral and verbal evidence for emotion, the pediatrician responds, "Yes, I can see that you are concerned." Which of the following statements would be the physician's best response?

    (A) "What in particular about this worries you?"
    (B) "I doubt that this is anything very serious."
    (C) "Has your daughter complained of burning when she goes to the bathroom?"
    (D) "This sometimes is a reflection of tension in the home."
    (E) "Symptoms like this can be alarming."

40. After the above conversation, the physician learns that the daughter has had no complaints of urinary tract infections, has been healthy previously, has been doing well in school, enjoys playing with several playmates, has a younger sister 5 years of age, and recently was very excited about the pending arrival of another sister. She seemed disappointed 1 week ago when her mother returned home from the hospital with a baby boy. Given this information, which of the following is the most likely diagnosis?

    (A) Adjustment disorder
    (B) Age-appropriate behavior
    (C) Conduct disorder
    (D) Functional enuresis
    (E) Occult cystitis

**41.** Assume that the diagnosis is supported during the initial visit with additional evidence after evaluation of the mother and the daughter. Which of the following actions would then be most appropriate therapeutically?

(A) Referral of the mother for psychological evaluation and possible individual psychotherapy

(B) Referral of the child for psychological evaluation and possible individual psychotherapy

(C) Referral of the child to a urologist for further diagnostic evaluation

(D) Referral of the child for psychological evaluation and behavioral therapy

(E) Educational psychotherapy by the pediatrician for the mother

*Questions 42–46*

*When answering this group of questions, you will need to refer to the 10 photographs in Chapter 2.*

Assume that you are a primary case physician working in an emergency department and that you have been summoned to take care of a boy, age 7 years, who has fallen off his bicycle. The boy has suffered a fracture of his right humerus. You have determined that the injury is a fracture by examining the boy and from a radiograph. In addition, the radiograph reveals that the fracture is through an area in which there is a benign cyst of the bone. Instead of the usual mobilization procedure, a consultation with an orthopedic surgeon will be necessary because surgery may be indicated. The charge nurse has determined the name of the boy's parents, who have been called. The father, Mr. Canfield, is the first to arrive.

You introduce yourself to Mr. Canfield and continue, "I think you may already know that your son, David, has been in an accident. (The father's face at this point appears similar to Photograph 5.) We've conducted an examination, have taken some x-rays, and have determined the extent of his injuries." (The father's face now appears similar to Photograph 6.)

42. Given the evidence and the early steps in the model of the therapeutic sequence, what is your correct response to Mr. Canfield?

    (A) "You're angry about something?"
    (B) "You're anxious to learn how your son is?"
    (C) "You're determined to know how your son is?"
    (D) "You seem surprised. Has no one told you?"
    (E) "Let me assure you, we have everything under control."

**43.** Assume that instead of the above sequence, at the end of your last statement, Mr. Canfield's face appears similar to Photograph 5. Given the circumstance, what is your response?

   **(A)** "You're angry about something?"
   **(B)** "You're anxious to know how your son is?"
   **(C)** "You're determined to know how your son is?"
   **(D)** "You seem surprised. Has no one told you?"
   **(E)** "Let me assure you, we have everything under control."

**44.** Assume that Mr. Canfield nods, acknowledging your response with a short, confirming response. You continue, "Your son has broken his right arm, the humerus bone, just below his right shoulder." (The father's face fleetingly appears similar to Photograph 3.) "Otherwise, he is all right judging from what we can tell from our examination." Mr. Canfield replies, "I suppose this means that he's going to need a cast and wear his arm in a sling for a while like I did when I broke my arm when I was a kid." (Mr. Canfield's face appears similar to Photograph 7.) You respond

   **(A)** "I guess you're feeling a little disgusted."
   **(B)** "I guess you're feeling a little disgusted, but I'm sure things will work out."
   **(C)** "I guess you're feeling disappointed."
   **(D)** "I guess you're feeling disappointed, but I'm sure he'll recover completely."
   **(E)** "I guess you're feeling a little upset."

**45.** Assume that Mr. Canfield replies to your statement confirming your observation and that you respond appropriately. Mr. Canfield continues, "But go on with whatever else you need to tell me." You continue, "This is an unusual fracture in some ways. It is called a pathologic fracture because the fracture occurred in a weakened place in the bone through a bone cyst. A bone cyst is a hollowed-out place in the bone that occurs in some people and makes the bone more liable to fracture. We certainly don't see evidence anywhere else in the x-rays for such cysts. I know that you're going to have a lot of questions about this, but let me tell you two things. First, your son will need to see a specialist, an orthopedic surgeon, to evaluate this situation, and second, nothing at the moment suggests that there is anything terribly serious going on in the cyst itself." (With the initial statement about the cyst, the patient's face looked similar to Photograph 3. However, at this point, assume that Mr. Canfield's face appears similar to Photograph 5.) Therefore, your response will most likely be

   **(A)** "You seem uneasy. Let me assure you that your son will get the best care."
   **(B)** "I know this is unexpected. You seem concerned. Is there a particular question?"
   **(C)** "I know this is unexpected. You seem concerned and that's understandable, but don't worry."
   **(D)** "You looked surprised. Now you seem relieved. You expected something more serious?"
   **(E)** "You looked surprised. Now you seem relieved. I guess you are afraid the cyst might have been cancer or something like that?"

**46.** Instead of the patient's face in the previous question looking similar to Photograph 5, assume that Mr. Canfield's face looks similar to Photograph 1. Given that information, what is your response?

(A) "You seem uneasy. Let me assure you that your son will get the best care."

(B) "I know this is unexpected. You seem concerned. Is there a particular question?"

(C) "I know this is unexpected. You seem concerned and that's understandable. Don't worry."

(D) "You look surprised. Now you seem relieved. You expected something more serious?"

(E) "You look surprised, even relieved. I guess you were afraid the cyst might have been cancer or something like that?"

DIRECTIONS: Each set of matching questions in this section consists of a list of four to twenty-six lettered options followed by several numbered items. For each numbered item, select the appropriate lettered option(s). Each lettered option may be selected once, more than once, or not at all. EACH ITEM WILL STATE THE NUMBER OF OPTIONS TO SELECT. CHOOSE EXACTLY THIS NUMBER.

*Questions 47–50*

    (A) Avoidant
    (B) Compulsive
    (C) Dependent
    (D) Histrionic
    (E) Narcissistic

Match each description below with the personality disorder that most closely matches it.

47. Most prone to psychophysiologic disorders (**SELECT ONE OPTION**)

48. Most prone to anxiety disorders (**SELECT ONE OPTION**)

49. Most prone to depressive disorders (**SELECT ONE OPTION**)

50. Most prone to substance abuse disorders (**SELECT ONE OPTION**)

*Questions 51–55*

   **(A)** Drowsiness, especially subject to psychological addiction
   **(B)** Dry mouth, akathisia
   **(C)** Dry mouth, hyperhidrosis
   **(D)** Hypertensive crisis with ingestion of foods high in tyramine
   **(E)** Polyuria, fine hand tremor

Match each of the following agents with the adverse effect that is most likely to occur from use of the drug.

51. Phenelzine sulfate (Nardil) (**SELECT ONE OPTION**)

52. Imipramine (Tofranil) (**SELECT ONE OPTION**)

53. Lithium carbonate (Eskalith) (**SELECT ONE OPTION**)

54. Diazepam (Valium) (**SELECT ONE OPTION**)

55. Chlorpromazine (Thorazine) (**SELECT ONE OPTION**)

*Questions 56–60*

    **(A)** Conversion disorder
    **(B)** Dissociative disorder
    **(C)** Generalized anxiety disorder (anxiety neurosis)
    **(D)** Major depression
    **(E)** Schizophrenia, paranoid type

For each of the following, assume the presence of a given illness and match it with the psychiatric disorder most likely to be *missed* as a superimposed disease.

**56.** Multiple sclerosis (**SELECT ONE OPTION**)

**57.** Mitral valve prolapse syndrome (**SELECT ONE OPTION**)

**58.** Temporal lobe epilepsy (**SELECT ONE OPTION**)

**59.** Hypothyroidism (**SELECT ONE OPTION**)

**60.** Phencyclidine abuse (**SELECT ONE OPTION**)

*Questions 61–65*

   (A) Conversion
   (B) Displacement
   (C) Introversion
   (D) Projection
   (E) Reaction formation

Match each diagnosis below with the defense mechanism characteristic of each.

61. Schizophrenic disorder, paranoid type (**SELECT ONE OPTION**)

62. Phobic disorder (**SELECT ONE OPTION**)

63. Obsessive–compulsive disorder (**SELECT ONE OPTION**)

64. Psychogenic pain disorder (**SELECT ONE OPTION**)

65. Major depression with melancholia (**SELECT ONE OPTION**)

*Questions 66–70*

**(A)** Eugene Bleuler
**(B)** James Braid
**(C)** Sigmund Freud
**(D)** Johann Weyer
**(E)** Erik Erikson

For each contribution listed below, match the name of the person associated with it.

66. Father of psychiatry (**SELECT ONE OPTION**)

67. Introduced the term "schizophrenia" (**SELECT ONE OPTION**)

68. Coined the term "hypnosis" (**SELECT ONE OPTION**)

69. Elaborated the concept of defense mechanisms (**SELECT ONE OPTION**)

70. Emphasized cultural influences in human behavior (**SELECT ONE OPTION**)

*Questions 71–75*

   (A)  Autistic thinking
   (B)  Clang association
   (C)  Concrete thinking
   (D)  Logical thinking
   (E)  Neologism

In an ambulatory setting, a physician asks a 25-year-old man, "What brings you to see me?" The patient responds with a series of statements. Match each of the following statements with the most appropriate diagnosis.

   71.  "A Ford." (**SELECT ONE OPTION**)

   72.  "A fine, flashy Ford, my lord." (**SELECT ONE OPTION**)

   73.  "You'd understand if your stomach made as much gas as mine does." (**SELECT ONE OPTION**)

   74.  "I am an outstanding gasogenic member of *Homo sapiens*." (**SELECT ONE OPTION**)

   75.  "That sounds crazy, doesn't it?" (**SELECT ONE OPTION**)

*Questions 76–80*

- **(A)** Major depression with psychotic features
- **(B)** Panic attacks
- **(C)** Psychophysiologic disorder, neck/shoulder/arm syndrome
- **(D)** Schizophreniform disorder
- **(E)** Uncomplicated bereavement

Each of the following five patients has a different personality structure. The severe stress of a recent death of a parent causes each patient to decompensate. Considering the structure of each personality, match the personality disorder listed below with the appropriate response.

76. Borderline personality disorder (**SELECT ONE OPTION**)

77. Dependent personality disorder (**SELECT ONE OPTION**)

78. Compulsive personality disorder (**SELECT ONE OPTION**)

79. Histrionic personality disorder (**SELECT ONE OPTION**)

80. Genital character (**SELECT ONE OPTION**)

*Questions 81–85*

    **(A)** Avoidant disorder
    **(B)** Conduct disorder, aggressive undersocialized type
    **(C)** Separation anxiety disorder
    **(D)** Sleep terrors
    **(E)** Transient tic disorder

Assume that each of the following patients as an adult has the following diagnosis. Match each with the most likely diagnosis of a childhood disorder made when the patient was a child.

81. Antisocial personality disorder (**SELECT ONE OPTION**)

82. Phobic disorder, social phobia type (**SELECT ONE OPTION**)

83. Generalized anxiety disorder (**SELECT ONE OPTION**)

84. Conversion disorder (**SELECT ONE OPTION**)

85. Genital character (**SELECT ONE OPTION**)

*Questions 86–90*

(A) Bipolar disorder, depressed phase
(B) Bipolar disorder, manic phase
(C) Dysthymic disorder
(D) Primary degenerative dementia, senile onset
(E) Schizophrenia, undifferentiated type

During a formal mental status examination, a physician asks a series of patients the following question: "What does this proverb mean to you: 'The grass is always greener on the other side of the street'?" Consider the responses. Although a single response to a proverb is not conclusive, given the following choices, match each with the most likely diagnosis.

86. "That means when you look across the street, the grass looks greener." (**SELECT ONE OPTION**)

87. "Well, Doc, sometimes that's true. If you know where to look, you can make a mint, and I'm on my way to a fortune. If you put some of your money in with me, I'll make you a millionaire." (**SELECT ONE OPTION**)

88. "I don't know." (**SELECT ONE OPTION**)

89. "Green is not my color." (**SELECT ONE OPTION**)

90. "That's the story of my life. No matter what I've done, on my side of the street, so to speak, it seems like there's been nothin' but bad luck. Of course, it's all my fault, I realize." (**SELECT ONE OPTION**)

*For Questions 91–110 you will need to review the following information and continue to refer to its details as you answer each question in this group.*

Consider the following five patients, all being seen for the first time by a family physician. In each instance, the physician makes the observations noted. The patient is making an opening statement.

*Mrs. Alport*, age 42. Average weight. Neat but old-fashioned dress. Sitting comfortably with hands in her lap. She speaks with a hint of whine in her voice. "Well, Doctor, I hardly know where to begin. I don't think I've had a well day in my life since I was in high school. I guess the worst are these excruciating headaches. Half the time I can't even fix meals, but my husband and children try to take care me. It's all very upsetting. They do the best they can, but I get annoyed and irritable sometimes because I don't think they realize how much I suffer! But then I have these dizzy spells and also have bowel trouble. Unless I'm very careful with what I eat I get sick to my stomach, and my periods have never been right."

*Mr. Brazil*, age 19. Dressed in red sport shirt and white slacks. Sitting with right leg crossed over left. He speaks with considerable inflection. "Well, there's nothing serious. I don't know why my parents are so concerned. I have this little headache." (Patient smiles.) "It's right here most of the time"; (he gestures dramatically with his right hand to an area about 5 to 6 cm in diameter over his right ear). "As you can see, I don't like to touch it because it's sensitive and shoots pains. Sometimes, it's kinda numb, though."

*Mr. Cooper*, age 54. Dressed in a conservative, expensive suit. Sitting with his right hand in a fist resting on the arm of the chair. Eyebrows are knit. Forehead is in a scowl. He speaks in a quiet and controlled manner. "I'll be brief. For 4 $\frac{1}{2}$ years, almost on a daily basis, mainly at work—I'm Vice President of the First National Bank, in charge of the loan division—beginning at noon, becoming severe in the late afternoon, I develop rather painful bilateral frontal headaches. I'll be frank with you. You are the third physician with whom I've consulted. I have not been satisfied with my experience in seeking relief from this malady to date." (With the last statement, he points his finger toward the physician.)

*Mrs. Duncan*, age 37. Dressed in skirt and blouse. Hands fidget somewhat. The patient looks at the physician with wide-open eyes and says, "Doctor, I'm frightened. For the last 2 weeks, I have been waking up early in the morning with a kind of a dull, throbbing headache mainly over my right eye. I've had headaches before but nothing like these, and this morning while reading the newspaper I happened to shut one eye and I noticed that the print was blurred, especially with my left eye closed."

*Mr. Eagleton*, age 41. Sitting in a rumpled sport coat. Hair uncombed. Head and eyes downcast, looking toward the floor. He speaks quietly and with little inflection. "Well, Doctor, I need help, but I don't think anybody can help me. I know I have to do it myself, but I can't seem to pull myself together since I got laid off at work, almost 1 year ago now. My wife is very understanding. I don't deserve her. She'd be better off without me. I just sit home and hardly want to get up. To be honest, I'm just awfully discouraged. I feel awful. I don't know what's going to become of me."

*Questions 91–95*

   (A)  Evidence for anxiety
   (B)  Evidence for anger
   (C)  Evidence for sadness
   (D)  Evidence for disgust
   (E)  Little evidence for any of the above, either
        objective or subjective

Match each patient with the appropriate emotion.

**91.** Mrs. Alport (**SELECT ONE OPTION**)

**92.** Mr. Brazil (**SELECT ONE OPTION**)

**93.** Mr. Cooper (**SELECT ONE OPTION**)

**94.** Mrs. Duncan (**SELECT ONE OPTION**)

**95.** Mr. Eagleton (**SELECT ONE OPTION**)

*Questions 96–100*

*Remember to refer to information presented in Questions 91–95 concerning these patients.*

(A) Conversion disorder
(B) Major depression
(C) Meningioma
(D) Musculotension headache
(E) Somatization disorder (Briquet's syndrome)

Match each patient below with the most likely diagnosis. A given answer should be used *only once*.

**96.** Mrs. Alport (**SELECT ONE OPTION**)

**97.** Mr. Brazil (**SELECT ONE OPTION**)

**98.** Mr. Cooper (**SELECT ONE OPTION**)

**99.** Mrs. Duncan (**SELECT ONE OPTION**)

**100.** Mr. Eagleton (**SELECT ONE OPTION**)

*Questions 101–105*

*Remember to refer to information presented in Questions 91–95 concerning these patients.*

  (A) Compulsive character
  (B) Dependent character
  (C) Genital character
  (D) Histrionic character
  (E) Narcissistic character

Match each patient below with the most likely character structure. A given answer should be used *only once*.

**101.** Mrs. Alport (**SELECT ONE OPTION**)

**102.** Mr. Brazil (**SELECT ONE OPTION**)

**103.** Mr. Cooper (**SELECT ONE OPTION**)

**104.** Mrs. Duncan (**SELECT ONE OPTION**)

**105.** Mr. Eagleton (**SELECT ONE OPTION**)

*Questions 106-110*

*Remember to refer to information presented in Questions 91-95 concerning these patients.*

(A) Noting neither objective nor subjective evidence for a distressing emotion when it would be expected, the physician inquires how the patient is feeling about his or her symptom

(B) Noting congruence of objective and subjective evidence, the physician acknowledges the emotion and formulates a question in an attempt to identify the category of stress

(C) Noting subjective evidence for an emotion but without objective evidence, the physician inquires whether the patient is feeling that way right now, intending then to confront the patient with the absence of objective evidence

(D) Noting objective evidence but an absence of subjective evidence, the physician inquires how the patient is feeling about the symptom and the situation just expressed

(E) Noting congruence between objective and subjective evidence and already sensing a consensus regarding the stress, the physician inquires what in particular the patient is distressed about

Recall that objective evidence refers to behavioral data and subjective evidence to verbal data. For each patient, identify the most appropriate question that the physician should ask in the interview.

**106.** Mrs. Alport (**SELECT ONE OPTION**)

**107.** Mr. Brazil (**SELECT ONE OPTION**)

**108.** Mr. Cooper (**SELECT ONE OPTION**)

**109.** Mrs. Duncan (**SELECT ONE OPTION**)

**110.** Mr. Eagleton (**SELECT ONE OPTION**)

*Questions 111–115*

(A) Avoidant behavioral response pattern
(B) Compulsive behavioral response pattern
(C) Histrionic behavioral response pattern
(D) Paranoid behavioral response pattern
(E) Schizoid behavioral response pattern

Match each patient described below with the most appropriate behavioral pattern. A given answer should be used *only once*.

111. Patient most likely to respond to frustration with anger with congruence between subjective and objective evidence (**SELECT ONE OPTION**)

112. Patient most likely to bring a malpractice suit against the health professional (**SELECT ONE OPTION**)

113. Patient most likely to be consistently late for appointments but always offers apologies (**SELECT ONE OPTION**)

114. Patient most likely to use the shortest sentences in answering questions (**SELECT ONE OPTION**)

115. The patient most likely to exhibit typical defense mechanisms that include rationalization, intellectualization, and reaction formation (**SELECT ONE OPTION**)

*Questions 116–130 all relate to the same five patients. Therefore, it is important that you keep in mind evidence regarding each patient as you answer each group of questions.*

*Questions 116–120*

- **(A)** Objective evidence for anxiety
- **(B)** Objective evidence for anger
- **(C)** Objective evidence for sadness
- **(D)** Objective evidence does not point to any of the above emotions

Assume that you are working in a private medical practice and see the following patients sitting in your waiting room. For each description, match the emotion expressed by that particular patient.

116. *Mr. Victor*, approximately 30 years of age, average weight for his height, wearing sport shirt and slacks. Sitting in slouched position in chair with legs crossed at the ankles. Periodically sighs deeply. Eyes usually looking at the floor. Hands periodically tap out a restless rhythm on the arms of the chair. Occasionally looks up, glancing at wall clock with wide open eyes. (**SELECT TWO OPTIONS**)

117. *Ms. Waters*, approximately 45 years of age, may be a few pounds underweight, conservatively dressed in dark suit. Sits fairly stiffly and upright in chair with legs crossed at knees. Face wears frown. Lips thin. (**SELECT ONE OPTION**)

118. *Ms. Xenophon*, approximately 22 years of age, average weight, dressed in pants suit. Sits fairly comfortably in chair. Reading a magazine. Occasionally smiling and shifting posture, apparently in response to items seen or read in magazine. (**SELECT ONE OPTION**)

119. *Mr. Yannity*, approximately 60 years of age and 5 to 10 pounds overweight, dressed in a casual suit. Sitting on edge of chair. Glances frequently about room with raised eyebrows. Eyes blink rapidly. Hands holding on fairly tightly to chair. (**SELECT ONE OPTION**)

120. *Ms. Zanowski*, approximately 50 years of age, somewhat overweight, dressed in a plain dress, holding a handkerchief in right hand. Head tilted forward and looking into lap. Occasionally wipes eyes with handkerchief. (**SELECT ONE OPTION**)

*Questions 121–125*

*Remember to refer to information presented in Questions 116–120 concerning these patients.*

    **(A)**   Subjective evidence for anxiety
    **(B)**   Subjective evidence for anger
    **(C)**   Subjective evidence for sadness
    **(D)**   Subjective evidence is lacking for any of the above primary emotions

Assume that you approach each of the following patients, mention their name, introduce yourself, escort them to your office, and gesture toward the chair in which they are to sit. Match each patient described with the emotional response noted.

**121.** *Mr. Victor* nods in response to your introduction. He takes a fairly deep breath and at the height of the inspiration says, "Good morning." After being seated, he responds to your opening nod by saying (all the while looking at the floor), "I really don't know exactly why I'm here. I don't really think that you or anybody else can help me." He pauses, waiting for your response. (**SELECT ONE OPTION**)

**122.** *Ms. Waters* responds to your introduction with a smile but you note that her face continues to wear the frown. She says, "I'm pleased to meet you." In your office, she responds to your opening nod by saying in a somewhat clipped voice, "I'm hoping to have a very thorough examination and evaluation. I simply have not been feeling as I should and, although I've had these headaches for years, they are clearly more intense in recent months." (**SELECT ONE OPTION**)

**123.** *Ms. Xenophon* responds to your introduction with an open smile. She says, "How do you do?" In response to your opening nod in your office, she leans forward somewhat and says, "I don't have any complaints in particular. It's been some time since I've had an examination. And besides, I'm thinking of getting married." With the latter statement, she smiles and blushes slightly. (**SELECT ONE OPTION**)

124. *Mr. Yannity* responds to your introduction by standing quickly, nodding, and saying, "Good morning." He walks rapidly down the hall. In your office, even before you are seated, he says, "Thank God you were able to see me so soon. I'm pretty nervous, I guess frightened would be a better word, about all this. Anyhow, for the last 2 or 3 days, I've noticed some bright red blood when I cough. I've had a cough for years, but I've never seen blood before." With this, he coughs gently and, with his right hand, strokes the back of his head. (**SELECT ONE OPTION**)

125. *Ms. Zanowski* responds to your introduction by simply nodding and rising slowly. In response to your opening nod in your office, she begins to weep. After a few moments, she attempts to control herself and says, "I'm sorry. I'm having a lot of trouble with myself. I apologize." (**SELECT ONE OPTION**)

*Questions 126–130*

*Remember to refer to information presented in Questions 116–120 concerning these patients.*

 (A) Injury or threat of injury
 (B) Frustration of drive or drive derivatives
 (C) Loss or threat of loss
 (D) Evidence to this point does not indicate clearly
  any of the above psychological stresses

Consider all of the available evidence presented to this point concerning these patients. Furthermore, assume that the evidence for emotion in any of the preceding patients corresponds with the usual or the expected category of psychological stress. Match the patient listed below with the category of stress.

**126.** Mr. Victor (**SELECT TWO OPTIONS**)

**127.** Ms. Waters (**SELECT ONE OPTION**)

**128.** Ms. Xenophon (**SELECT ONE OPTION**)

**129.** Mr. Yannity (**SELECT ONE OPTION**)

**130.** Ms. Zanowski (**SELECT ONE OPTION**)

*Questions 131–150 all relate to the same five patients. Therefore, it is important that you keep in mind evidence regarding each patient as you answer each of the following questions.*

*Questions 131–135*

    **(A)** Objective evidence for anxiety
    **(B)** Objective evidence for anger
    **(C)** Objective evidence for sadness
    **(D)** Objective evidence does not point to any of the above emotions

Match each patient described below with the appropriate emotion.

131. *Ms. Alvarado.* Age 23. Appearance is thin, even gaunt. Dressed in skirt and shirt blouse. Sits relatively comfortably in chair in waiting room. Seems to be looking at a painting on the wall. Relatively immobile, ignores conversation of other patients. (**SELECT ONE OPTION**)

132. *Mr. Mundt.* Age 19. Average weight. Dressed in T-shirt and jeans. Sits with back resting against the back of the chair. Appears tense. Legs tightly crossed. Scowling facial demeanor. (**SELECT ONE OPTION**)

133. *Mrs. Santos.* Age 50. Somewhat overweight. Dressed neatly in plain dress and jewelry. Sits in somewhat slumped position in chair. Eyes are cast downward toward the floor. Hand grasps a handkerchief. (**SELECT ONE OPTION**)

134. *Mr. Crockett.* Age 24. Average weight. Dressed in sport shirt and slacks. Patient is standing, leaning against the wall. Face is relatively expressionless. Seems to be chatting somewhat uncomfortably with Ms. Jules. (**SELECT ONE OPTION**)

135. *Ms. Jules.* Age 34. Average weight. Attractively dressed in a pants suit. Occasionally rubs her forehead above her right eye. Sitting somewhat forward in the chair. Licks lips several times when talking with Mr. Crockett. (**SELECT ONE OPTION**)

*Questions 136–140*

*Remember to refer to information presented in Questions 131–135 concerning these patients.*

(A)  Subjective evidence for anxiety, anger, or sadness is present. Subjective evidence is incongruent with objective evidence

(B)  Subjective evidence for anxiety, anger, or sadness is present. Subjective evidence is congruent with objective evidence

(C)  Subjective evidence for anxiety, anger, or sadness is absent. Subjective evidence is congruent with objective evidence

(D)  Subjective evidence for anxiety, anger, or sadness is absent. Subjective evidence is incongruent with objective evidence

Match each of the following patients with the appropriate diagnosis.

**136.** *Ms. Alvarado.* Patient sits comfortably in the chair. Glances at you briefly and responds to your opening nod by saying rather quietly, "I have these headaches all the time. They're making me so nervous I can hardly stand it much longer." She pauses, then adds, "I've had them for years." She stops at this point, waiting for your response. (**SELECT ONE OPTION**)

**137.** *Mr. Mundt.* Patient moves vigorously into your office and sits down briskly. He continues to scowl when looking at you and responds to your opening nod as follows. "I'm having these headaches right here in front, and I've been having them for quite a few months now, no matter where I go. I think it must be allergies or something. Anyhow, I want you to give me something so they won't be such a drag." (**SELECT ONE OPTION**)

138. *Mrs. Santos.* Patient walks slowly into the room. After a long sigh, she responds to your opening nod, "I'm feeling so discouraged. I keep having these headaches. I've had them for at least the last 6 months. Sometimes I have trouble going to sleep." She pauses for a few moments, you remain silent, and she continues, "I guess that's mainly because I lay there worrying about all the things I have to do. I used to be a very good housekeeper, but since my husband died, I guess I don't have quite the motivation I used to have." (**SELECT ONE OPTION**)

139. *Mr. Crockett.* After the patient is seated, he responds to your opening nod by saying in a rather bland manner, "My wife thought I ought to see you. She's concerned about this pain I have in my head. It's right here on the left side. The spot is about as big as my hand. (He gestures with his left hand delineating the left parietal area.) I think she's wondering whether it's a brain tumor or something like that. I keep telling her it's nothing to be concerned about." (**SELECT ONE OPTION**)

140. *Ms. Jules.* After being seated, Ms. Jules fidgets a bit with her hands and responds to your opening nod by saying, "I notice I'm a little nervous today and, to tell the truth, I've been anxious for the past week or so. For the first time in my life I have a headache, and it doesn't seem to go away. Last night I really had trouble sleeping. Until now, I didn't know what a headache was. I wonder if it's because I'm under some sort of pressure. I sometimes do get a little anxious about that, but I've never had a headache like this." (**SELECT ONE OPTION**)

*Questions 141–145*

*Remember to refer to information presented in Questions 131–135 concerning these patients.*

(A)  Avoidant behavioral response pattern
(B)  Compulsive behavioral response pattern
(C)  Genital character
(D)  Narcissistic behavioral response pattern
(E)  Schizoid behavioral response pattern

Given the available evidence concerning each patient, match each patient described below with the most likely diagnosis.

**141.** Ms. Alvarado (**SELECT ONE OPTION**)

**142.** Mr. Mundt (**SELECT ONE OPTION**)

**143.** Mrs. Santos (**SELECT ONE OPTION**)

**144.** Mr. Crockett (**SELECT ONE OPTION**)

**145.** Ms. Jules (**SELECT ONE OPTION**)

*Questions 146–150*

*Remember to refer to information presented in Questions 131–135 concerning these patients.*

(A) Conversion reaction
(B) Referred pain secondary to an apical abscess of an upper molar
(C) Headaches beginning in occipital region, muscular-type tension, origin psychophysiologic
(D) Headaches beginning in frontal region, muscular-type tension, origin psychophysiologic
(E) Headaches poorly described, generalized throughout head, origin psychosomatic, most likely related to depression

Given the available evidence, match each patient listed below with the most likely diagnosis.

146. Ms. Alvarado (**SELECT ONE OPTION**)

147. Mr. Mundt (**SELECT ONE OPTION**)

148. Mrs. Santos (**SELECT ONE OPTION**)

149. Mr. Crockett (**SELECT ONE OPTION**)

150. Ms. Jules (**SELECT ONE OPTION**)

## PSYCHIATRY AND BEHAVIORAL MEDICINE ANSWERS AND DISCUSSION

**1–E (Preface)** This question and questions 2 and 3 will indicate something about how you understand this review book and perhaps even something about how you will read and learn from it.

**2–There is no *correct* answer (Preface)** Physicians, as a group, are highest on the economic scale, with the political scale being second. Individual physicians vary considerably (remember this is not a profile of values. Physicians are ranked among the highest for measures of altruism). Characteristic of genital characters is that they know their need profile. Then comes the question, "How do I structure my practice to gratify my needs but remain within the bounds of my professional ethics and commitment to my patients?" Physicians will resist change, like any other group, when their psychological need profile is challenged.

**3–Answers will vary (Preface)** Many physicians are discomfited when asked to look at themselves. Others are pleased with the opportunity.

**4–D (Chapter 1; Table 1-1)** The biopsychosocial model suggests that the expected emotional and behavioral response to the category of stress termed "the unexpected" would be surprise and orienting behavior.

**5–E (Chapter 1)** Approximately 25% to 30% of visits to ambulatory care medical facilities can be attributed directly to mental illness.

**6–B (Chapter 2)** This surgeon expects *every* patient to be anxious.

**7–A (Chapter 2)** The individual response specificity states that before the response of a given human to a given stimulus can be predicted, the individual must first be understood.

**8–E (Chapter 2; Table 2-1)** As can be seen in Table 2-1, tobacco is the leading actual cause of death in the United States.

**9–D (Chapter 2)** The physician has identified the primary emotion exhibited in this patient, and an efficient and effective response to this patient would be for the physician to identify that the patient is feeling slightly anxious.

**10–B (Chapter 2)** Of significance in the evaluation of this patient is obtaining a description of behavior from someone in addition to the mother.

**11–A (Chapter 2)** Delta activity is not characteristic of a convulsive disorder.

**12–C (Chapter 3)** The largest group of cases of mental retardation, approximately 30% of the patient population, is termed *primary*. This designates those instances in which no specific etiology can be identified or be reasonably postulated. Perinatal infections, especially viral and early childhood encephalitides, cause about 20% of cases. Prematurity and birth trauma may account for another 20%. Down's syndrome is common.

**13–C (Chapter 3)** Patients with anorexia frequently report feeling fat when they are emaciated. Anorexia is essentially self-induced starvation and occurs more often in adolescent girls than in adolescent boys.

**14–A (Chapter 3)** The etiology does not speak to biogenesis.

**15–A (Chapter 4)** Clouding of consciousness, which is absent in schizophrenia, is typical of delirium.

**16–D (Chapter 4)** Note the withdrawal symptoms associated with delirium tremens, or alcohol withdrawal syndrome.

**17–A (Chapter 4)** Approximately 5% to 15% of people older than 65 years of age have Alzheimer's-type dementia.

**18–C (Chapter 4)** Cocaine does not produce a withdrawal syndrome; the other substances listed produce withdrawal syndromes.

**19–B (Chapter 4)** Intoxication caused by amphetamines is most likely to be confused with an acute schizophrenic disorder.

**20–C (Chapter 4)** Depression is not a typical feature of delirium.

**21–D (Chapter 5)** About 1% to 3% of the population is affected by schizophrenia.

**22–D (Chapter 7)** A genetic component is least compelling in panic disorder.

**23–D (Chapter 14)** Patients with bipolar disorder may have an acute episode precipitated by use of imipramine (Tofranil).

**24–E (Chapter 6)** Many patients who present in ambulatory primary care settings with complaints suggesting depression do not fall into any diagnostic category. These patients speak of themselves as "depressed," and have experienced losses and are responding appropriately to grief as uncomplicated bereavement.

**25–B (Chapter 14)** The preferred treatment for panic disorder is with a tricyclic antidepressant such as imipramine, which has an inhibiting effect presumably at the level of the locus ceruleus.

**26–B (Chapter 14)** Desipramine (Norpramin) is the drug of choice for this patient diagnosed with a major depression with psychotic features, who has been treated with imipramine but has not responded. If patients do not respond to one class of tricyclic agents, they may respond to another.

**27–E (Chapter 9)** This patient has sexual arousal disorder, characterized by reported sexual interest but partial or complete failure to attain or maintain erection throughout the sex act.

**28–A (Chapter 11)** Psychological factors are often prominent in dermatitis factitia, hyperhidrosis, rosacea, and urticaria, but do not affect acne.

**29–A (Chapter 11)** The term "dermatitis factitia" implies a lesion created by the patient.

**30–D (Chapter 14)** Situations that require special consideration when using electroconvulsive therapy are if the patient has an aortic aneurysm or coronary artery disease, detached retina, brain tumor, or increased intracranial pressure, is pregnant, or has bone and joint disease, but these are not absolute contraindications *per se*.

**31–D (Chapter 14)** When therapists involve patients in the problem-solving process, compliance is enhanced.

**32–B (Chapter 14)** Transference refers to the unconscious tendency of the patient to respond to the therapist as if he or she were someone else, such as a significant other in the patient's present or past.

**33–E (Chapter 2)** Men are taught not to display sadness; therefore, they tend not to see sadness in other men.

**34–A (Chapter 14)** By saying nothing but using nonverbal indicators, the patient is encouraged to follow her train of thought.

**35–A (Chapter 14)** A specific communication problem between two people suggests a modality of therapy best suited to that problem.

**36–B (Chapter 2)** The patient says directly that he is discouraged, and the description of his nonverbal behavior is classic for sadness.

**37–D (Chapter 2)** The patient is incongruent for sadness. Attempting to identify the stress is the next step.

**38–B (Chapter 6)** Compare the evidence in the patient with the description in the text of a major depressive disorder.

**39–A (Chapter 2)** The mother is congruent for anxiety. The physician proceeds to identify the stress.

**40–B (Chapter 3)** This is an example of age-appropriate behavior.

**41–E (Chapter 14)** The mother needs to know that such a response is common in this situation and does not indicate a serious pathologic process. Therefore, the most appropriate action would be educational psychotherapy by the pediatrician for the mother.

**42–C (Chapter 2 and Appendix)** Although objective evidence points to anger, "determined" is a better choice and less likely to encourage an adverse response.

**43–B (Chapter 2 and Appendix)** His face suggests anxiety. You ask directly to obtain congruence.

**44–C (Chapter 2 and Appendix)** His face suggests sadness (disappointed); answer (D) involves premature reassurance.

**45–B (Chapter 2 and Appendix)** The process has led to congruence for anxiety. A question to determine the particular concern is in order.

**46–D (Chapter 2 and Appendix)** Following the face of surprise comes the face of acceptance. A question to determine what was surprising is most appropriate.

**47–B (Chapter 12)** The person with a compulsive personality disorder is most likely to suffer from psychophysiologic disorders.

**48–D (Chapter 12)** The person with a histrionic personality disorder is most prone to development of anxiety disorders.

**49–A (Chapter 12)** A person with avoidant personality disorders is most likely to manifest depressive disorders.

**50–C (Chapter 12)** The person with a dependent personality disorder is most likely vulnerable to substance abuse.

**51–D (Chapter 14)** Phenelzine sulfate is associated with adverse effects such as hypertensive crisis with ingestion of foods high in tyramine.

**52–C (Chapter 14)** Imipramine is associated with adverse effects such as dry mouth and hyperhidrosis.

**53–E (Chapter 14)** Long-term use of lithium carbonate is associated with polyuria, polydipsia, and fine hand tremor.

**54–A (Chapter 14)** Antianxiety agents such as diazepam are associated with drowsiness. Patients taking these agents are especially subject to psychological addiction. Long-term use tends to support the patients' tendencies to avoid facing their psychological problems and effecting more appropriate solutions.

**55–B (Chapter 14)** Dry mouth and akathisia are associated with the use of chlorpromazine.

**56–A (Chapter 8)** The diagnosis most likely to be missed as a superimposed disease is conversion disorder in the presence of multiple sclerosis.

**57–C (Chapters 8 and 11)** The diagnosis most likely to be missed as a superimposed disease is generalized anxiety disorder (anxiety neurosis) in the presence of mitral valve prolapse syndrome.

**58–B (Chapter 8)** The diagnosis most likely to be missed as a superimposed disease is a dissociative disorder in the presence of temporal lobe epilepsy.

**59–D (Chapter 6)** The diagnosis most likely to be missed as a superimposed disease is major depression in the presence of hypothyroidism.

**60–E (Chapter 4)** The diagnosis most likely to be missed as a superimposed disease is schizophrenia, paranoid type in the presence of phencyclidine abuse. In each case in questions 56–60, note the similarity of symptoms.

**61–D (Chapter 5)** The diagnosis is schizophrenic disorder, paranoid type—the defense mechanism is projection.

**62–B (Chapter 7)** The diagnosis is phobic disorder—the defense mechanism is displacement.

**63–E (Chapter 7)** The diagnosis is obsessive–compulsive disorder—the defense mechanism is reaction formation.

**64–A (Chapter 8)** The diagnosis is psychogenic pain disorder—the defense mechanism is conversion.

**65–C (Chapter 6)** The diagnosis is major depression with melancholia—the defense mechanism is introversion.

**66–D (Chapter 1)** Johann Weyer is known as the father of psychiatry.

**67–A (Chapter 1)** Eugene Bleuler introduced the term "schizophrenia."

**68–B (Chapter 1)** James Braid coined the term "hypnosis."

**69–C (Chapter 1)** Sigmund Freud elaborated concepts such as defense mechanisms, the unconscious, ego, id, and superego, which have become an integral part of psychiatric thought.

**70–E (Chapter 1)** Erik Erikson emphasized cultural influences in human behavior.

**71–C (Chapter 5)** The phrase, "A Ford," is an example of concrete thinking.

**72–B (Chapter 5)** The statement, "A fine, flashy Ford, my lord," is an example of clang association.

**73–A (Chapter 5)** The statement, "You'd understand if your stomach made as much gas as mine does," is an example of autistic thinking.

**74–C (Chapter 5)** The statement, "I am an outstanding gasogenic member of *Homo sapiens*," is an example of concrete thinking.

**75–D (Chapter 5)** The statement, "That sounds crazy, doesn't it?" is an example of logical thinking. The entire series of statements in questions 71–75 was made by a patient with schizophrenia and exemplifies the thought disorder characteristic of the illness.

**76–D (Chapter 12)** When patients with borderline personality disorder are under profound stress, they regress profoundly and may appear psychotic.

**77–A (Chapter 12)** The patient with dependent personality disorder is very vulnerable to loss, and severe regression to depression is common.

**78–C (Chapter 12)** Patients with compulsive personality disorder "hide" their feeling responses from themselves and others; therefore, they respond through the body with a psychophysiologic disorder such as neck/shoulder/arm syndrome.

**79–B (Chapter 12)** A patient with a histrionic personality disorder often perceives a loss as a threat to self, evoking anxiety.

**80–E (Chapter 6)** Normal, nonneurotic people (genital characters) respond to loss with grief, uncomplicated bereavement.

**81–B (Chapters 3 and 12)** Note the similarity of behaviors in patients with antisocial personality disorder and conduct disorder, aggressive undersocialized type. People with conduct disorder are characterized as having a repetitive and persistent pattern of conduct for at least 6 months in which the basic rights of others are either ignored or violated. The behaviors may be aggressive (e.g., physical violence against property or people) or nonaggressive (e.g., a recurring and chronic tendency to violate rules or to lie). Antisocial personality disorder, when diagnosed in patients younger than 15 years of age, is characterized, for example, by truancy, behavioral delinquency, persistent lying, casual sexual intercourse, substance abuse, and initiation of fights. After age 18 years, the manifestations of the disorder include an inability to sustain consistent work behavior, inability to function in a consistent manner as a responsible parent, failure to accept social norms with respect to lawful behavior, and disregard for the truth as indicated by lying.

**82–A (Chapters 3 and 12)** Consider the dynamics of avoidant disorder in children; hence, displacement and phobias manifest in adults. Phobias often have their onset in childhood and adolescence. Avoidant personality disorder is characterized by hypersensitivity to rejection, an unwillingness to enter into relationships unless given strong guarantees of uncritical acceptance, social withdrawal, a desire for affection, and usually by extremely low self-esteem.

**83–C (Chapters 3 and 7)** Note the similarity in symptoms of the patient with generalized anxiety disorder and separation anxiety disorder. Generalized anxiety disorder is characterized by manifestations of anxiety either consistently present or frequently recurring. The patient may report a subjective awareness of this anxiety, using such expressions as fear, afraid, apprehension, worry, and so forth. Or, they may describe feeling constantly on the alert, dreading some unknown and unidentified danger or tragedy; or they may report various of the psychophysiologic manifestations of anxiety such as sweating, feeling cold, clammy hands, light-headedness, or a combination of symptoms. Separation anxiety disorder is an attachment disorder of infancy and childhood and is quite common. Patients experience excessive anxiety clearly relating to separation from a significant person to whom the child feels attached. Symptoms should be present for at least 2 weeks before this diagnosis is made.

**84–E (Chapters 3 and 7)** The childhood psychogenic tic disorder is repeated in adulthood with conversion musculoskeletal symptoms. Tics are characterized as recurrent, involuntary, repetitive, purposeless movements. A tic disorder may be subclassified as either transient (present for at least 1 month but no more than 1 year) or chronic. The syndrome usually is thought to be psychogenic in origin; hence counseling and psychotherapy are indicated. Conversion disorders are characterized by an involuntary psychogenic loss or disorder of function, often suggesting a physical illness.

**85–D (Chapter 3)** Sleep terrors are a developmental disorder, not psychogenic; therefore, they do not predict adult psychopathology.

**86–D (Chapter 4)** The patient with dementia suffers impairment of abstract thinking, with a return of concrete thinking.

**87–B (Chapter 6)** Note the suggestion of grandiosity, characteristic of the manic phase of bipolar disorder.

**88–A (Chapter 6)** With major depression, patients often seem to have little energy to think.

**89–E (Chapter 5)** The patient has schizophrenia, undifferentiated type; this is an autistic response.

**90–C (Chapter 6)** Symbolic thinking but a tendency to blame the self (introversion) is typical of patients with less severe depression, or dysthymic disorder.

**91–B (Chapter 2)** Mrs. Alport—the emotion is evidence for anger.

**92–E (Chapter 2)** Mr. Brazil—there is little evidence for any of the emotions, either objective or subjective.

**93–B (Chapter 2)** Mr. Cooper—the emotion is evidence for anger.

**94–A (Chapter 2)** Mrs. Duncan—the emotion is evidence for anxiety.

**95–C (Chapter 2)** Mr. Eagleton—the emotion is evidence for sadness.

**96–E (Chapter 8)** Mrs. Alport—the diagnosis is somatization disorder. Note the multiple complaints of the patient.

**97–A (Chapter 8)** Mr. Brazil—diagnosis is conversion disorder. Note the suggestion of *la belle indifférence*.

**98–D (Chapter 11)** Mr. Cooper—diagnosis is musculotension headache. Given the illness script, this is the most likely of the diagnoses.

**99–C (Chapter 2)** Mrs. Duncan—diagnosis is meningioma. The patient is congruent. The symptoms are recent and wake her up.

**100–B (Chapter 6)** Mr. Eagleton—diagnosis is major depression. The illness script presented by the patient most closely approximates this diagnosis.

**101–E (Chapter 12)** Mrs. Alport—narcissistic character.

**102–D (Chapter 12)** Mr. Brazil—histrionic character.

**103–A (Chapter 12)** Mr. Cooper—compulsive character.

**104–C (Chapter 12)** Mrs. Duncan—genital character.

**105–B (Chapter 12)** Mr. Eagleton—dependent character. The instance script presented by these patients most closely approximates the axis II diagnoses.

**106–C (Chapter 2)** The physician should ask Mrs. Alport whether she is feeling that way at the present, intending to confront her with the absence of objective evidence. There is subjective evidence.

**107–A (Chapter 2)** The physician should ask Mr. Brazil how he is feeling about his symptom because there is neither objective nor subjective evidence for a distressing emotion when it is expected.

**108–D (Chapter 2)** The physician should ask Mr. Cooper about the symptom and the situation just expressed; there is objective evidence but no subjective evidence.

**109–E (Chapter 2)** The physician should ask Mrs. Duncan specifically what is distressing to her.

**110–B (Chapter 2)** The physician should formulate a question attempting to identify the category of stress associated with Mr. Eagleton.

**111–C (Chapter 12)** The patient most likely to respond to frustration with anger with congruence between subjective and objective evidence exhibits a histrionic behavioral response pattern.

**112–D (Chapter 12)** The patient most likely to bring a malpractice suit against the health professional exhibits a paranoid behavioral response pattern.

**113–A (Chapter 12)** The patient most likely to be consistently late for appointments but who always offers apologies exhibits an avoidant behavioral response pattern.

**114–E (Chapter 12)** The patient most likely to use the shortest sentences in answering questions exhibits a schizoid behavioral response pattern.

**115–B (Chapter 12)** The patient most likely to use typical defense mechanisms, which include rationalization, intellectualization, and reaction formation exhibits a compulsive behavioral response pattern.

**116–B and C (Chapter 2 and Appendix)** Mr. Victor—the emotions expressed are objective evidence for anger and for sadness.

**117–B (Chapter 2 and Appendix)** Ms. Waters—the emotion is objective evidence for anger.

**118–D (Chapter 2 and Appendix)** Ms. Xenophon—objective evidence does not point to any of the above emotions.

**119–A (Chapter 2 and Appendix)** Mr. Yannity—the emotion expressed is objective evidence for anxiety.

**120–C (Chapter 2 and Appendix)** Ms. Zanowski—the emotion expressed is objective evidence for sadness.

**121–D (Chapter 2)** Mr. Victor—subjective evidence is lacking for any of the above primary emotions.

**122–D (Chapter 2)** Ms. Waters—subjective evidence is lacking for any of the above primary emotions.

**123–D (Chapter 2)** Mrs. Xenophon—subjective evidence is lacking for any of the primary emotions.

**124–A (Chapter 2)** Mr. Yannity—the emotional response is subjective evidence for anxiety.

**125–D (Chapter 2)** Ms. Zanowski—subjective evidence is lacking for any of the above primary emotions.

**126–A and B (Chapter 2)** Mr. Victor—the categories of stress are injury or threat of injury and frustration of drive or drive derivatives.

**127–B (Chapter 2)** Ms. Waters—the category of stress is frustration of drive or drive derivatives.

**128–D (Chapter 2)** Ms. Xenophon—there is no evidence at this point that indicates clearly any of the above psychological stresses.

**129–A (Chapter 2)** Mr. Yannity—the category of stress is injury or threat of injury.

**130–C (Chapter 2)** Ms. Zanowski—the category of stress is loss or threat of loss.

**131–D (Chapter 2)** Ms. Alvarado—the objective evidence does not point to any of the above emotions.

**132–B (Chapter 2)** Mr. Mundt—there is objective evidence that points to anger. The patient appears tense, has a scowling facial demeanor, and sits with his legs tightly crossed.

**133–C (Chapter 2)** Mrs. Santos—there is objective evidence that points to sadness. The patient sits in a somewhat slumped position in the chair with her eyes cast downward toward the floor. Her hand grasps a handkerchief.

**134–D (Chapter 2)** Mr. Crockett—the objective evidence does not point to any of the above emotions.

**135–A (Chapter 2)** Ms. Jules—there is objective evidence for anxiety. She occasionally rubs her forehead above her right eye and licks her lips several times while talking with another patient. She also sits forward in her chair.

**136–A (Chapter 2)** Ms. Alvarado—subjective evidence for anxiety, anger, or sadness is present. The subjective evidence is incongruent with objective evidence.

**137–D (Chapter 2)** Mr. Mundt—subjective evidence for anxiety, anger, or sadness is absent. The subjective evidence is incongruent with objective evidence.

**138–B (Chapter 2)** Mrs. Santos—subjective evidence for anxiety, anger, or sadness is present. The subjective evidence is congruent with objective evidence.

**139–C (Chapter 2)** Mr. Crockett—subjective evidence for anxiety, anger, or sadness is absent. The subjective evidence is incongruent with objective evidence.

**140–B (Chapter 2)** Ms. Jules—subjective evidence for anxiety, anger, or sadness is present. The subjective evidence is congruent with objective evidence.

**141–E (Chapter 12)** Ms. Alvarado—the diagnosis is schizoid behavioral response pattern. This type of personality is characterized by emotional coldness or aloofness, absence of tender feelings toward others, and by relative indifference to praise or criticism or to the feelings of others. Patients tend to have very few if any close friends but may be very attached to animals. They may have outstanding academic records, having spent hours alone studying. As adolescents, they tend to be seen as shy and withdrawn.

**142–D (Chapter 12)** Mr. Mundt—the diagnosis is narcissistic behavioral response pattern. People with this type of personality disorder possess a grandiose sense of self-importance or uniqueness and often are preoccupied with fantasies of unlimited success, power, brilliance, or beauty. There may be a quality of exhibitionism. Often they expect special favors from others without assuming reciprocity. They lack empathy and tend to relate to others by alternating between the extremes of overidealization and devaluation.

**143–B (Chapter 12)** Mrs. Santos—the diagnosis is compulsive behavioral response pattern. These people are preoccupied with details, rules, order, organization, schedules, and lists. They often are given, or give themselves, the appellation of *perfectionist*. Compulsive characters are rigid, lacking flexibility, and use defense mechanisms such as intellectualization, rationalization, compartmentalization, and reaction formation. These people seem fixated on a stage of life in which great emphasis is placed on doing things right so as to avoid punishment or shame.

**144–C (Chapter 12)** Mr. Crockett—the diagnosis is a genital character, or mixed personality disorder, in which people have features of more than one of the previously discussed disorders and do not meet the full criteria for a specific category. Genital characters may show features of any or all of the above personality disorders, but none of the patterns predominate or endure to the point such behavior becomes maladaptive to a given situation. Possibly 20% to 30% of the adult population may be genital characters.

**145–A (Chapter 12)** Ms. Jules—the diagnosis is avoidant behavioral response pattern. This character is typified by hypersensitivity to rejection, an unwillingness to enter into relationships unless given strong guarantees of uncritical acceptance. There is social withdrawal, a desire for affection, and usually extremely low self-esteem. They avoid confrontation. They often appear afraid of success but yet desperately seek success. Outwardly they may behave in a manner similar to the schizoid, but these people are afraid of the world's shame and ridicule.

**146–C (Chapters 11 and 12)** Mrs. Alvarado—the patient is diagnosed with headaches beginning in the occipital region, with muscular-type tension. The origin is psychophysiologic.

**147–D (Chapters 11 and 12)** Mr. Mundt—the patient is diagnosed with headaches beginning in the frontal region, muscular-type tension. The origin is psychophysiologic.

**148–E (Chapters 11 and 12)** Mrs. Santos—the patient is diagnosed with headaches poorly described, generalized throughout the head. The origin is psychosomatic, and is most likely related to depression.

**149–A (Chapters 8 and 12)** Mr. Crockett—the patient is diagnosed with conversion reaction, characterized by an involuntary psychogenic loss or disorder of function that often suggests a physical illness. Symptoms are typically limited to impairment of motor or sensory functions (e.g., blindness, paresthesia, paralysis), but they also may involve the autonomic nervous system to a lesser degree. Symptoms typically begin and end suddenly. Usually the symptoms resolve once the underlying conflict is resolved.

**150–B (Chapters 6 and 12)** Ms. Jules—the diagnosis is referred pain secondary to an apical abscess of an upper molar.

# Psychiatry and Behavioral Medicine
## Must-Know Topics

The following are must-know topics discussed in this review. It would be useful for you to formulate outlines on these subjects because knowledge of the related material will be key to your understanding of the subject and material and for passing the examination.

- Adjustment disorders

- Anxiety disorders: panic, generalized, obsessive–compulsive, posttraumatic stress disorder

- Cognitive impairments

- Delirium versus dementia; Alzheimer's disease; multi-infarct dementia

- Infancy, childhood, and adolescence: associated disorders, including attention deficit–hyperactivity, conduct disorder, anxiety disorder, adjustment reaction, eating disorders, movement and developmental disorders

- Metabolic and endocrine disorders

*(continued)*

- Mood disorders: major affective, major depressive, bipolar (manic–depressive), major depression (unipolar, endogenous), cyclothymic, dysthymic, bereavement, grief

- Personality disorders: schizotypal, paranoid, schizoid, antisocial, borderline, narcissistic, histrionic, dependent, compulsive, avoidant, mixed

- Schizophrenia; schizophreniform disorder; schizoaffective disorder

- Sexual and gender disorders: sexual dysfunction

- Somatoform disorders: Briquet's syndrome, conversion, pain, hypochondriasis, dissociative, multiple personality, depersonalization

- Substance abuse and dependence: cocaine, tobacco, alcohol, opioids, amphetamines, barbiturates, benzodiazepines; tolerance, withdrawal

- Treatment: psychotherapy, pharmacotherapy

▼

# Index

Page numbers followed by a *t* refer to tables; those followed by an *f* refer to figures.